THE

AUTOIMMUNE

PROTOCOL

Ethan Lawson

A Proven Guide to Autoimmune Disease, Restoring Gut Health, and Reclaiming Your Life Through Diet and Lifestyle Changes

©Ethan Lawson

2025. All rights reserved.

No part of this book may be reproduced, stored, or transmitted in any form or by any means, electronic, mechanical, photocopying, recording, scanning, or otherwise, except as permitted under Section 107 or 108 of the 1976 United States Copyright Act, without the prior written permission of the Publisher.

About the Author

Ethan Lawson is a passionate health advocate and expert in autoimmune diseases, with over 15 years of experience in the field of functional medicine. He has dedicated his career to helping individuals overcome chronic autoimmune conditions through evidence-based nutrition, lifestyle changes, and personalized care. After witnessing the transformative power of the Autoimmune Protocol (AIP) in his own life, Dr. Lawson began to share his knowledge with others, offering a path to healing that emphasizes the importance of diet, gut health, and holistic wellness.

Lawson holds a Doctorate in Medicine and has undergone specialized training in autoimmune disease management, nutrition, and integrative health practices. Throughout his career, he has helped hundreds of patients regain control of their health, using a combination of medical insights and cutting-edge dietary protocols.

In addition to his clinical practice, Lawson is a sought-after speaker and author, contributing to health publications and conducting seminars aimed at educating the public on autoimmune diseases and sustainable lifestyle solutions. His approach is rooted in compassion, research, and a deep understanding of how the body can heal when given the right tools.

Lawson's mission is to empower individuals to take charge of their autoimmune health and live vibrant, active lives free from the constraints of chronic illness. Through his book, *The Autoimmune Protocol*, he shares not only his expertise but also the stories of real people who have healed their bodies and transformed their lives with the power of AIP.

THE ROLE OF DIET AND LIFESTYLE IN AUTOIMMUNITY

Autoimmune diseases are a complex interplay of genetic predispositions, environmental triggers, and immune system dysfunction. While the precise cause of autoimmunity remains elusive, research has increasingly highlighted the critical role diet and lifestyle play in the onset, progression, and management of these conditions. Unlike conventional treatment approaches that often focus on symptom management through medications, diet and lifestyle interventions target the root causes of inflammation and immune system imbalances, offering a holistic pathway to improved health.

The Diet-Immune Connection

Diet is a foundational pillar in managing autoimmunity because it directly influences inflammation, gut health, and immune system activity. Certain foods are known to trigger inflammatory responses, exacerbating autoimmune symptoms. For instance, gluten, dairy, sugar, and processed foods are common culprits that can irritate the gut lining, leading to increased intestinal permeability—commonly referred to as "leaky gut." This condition allows undigested food particles, toxins, and pathogens to enter the bloodstream, triggering an immune response that can fuel autoimmune activity.

Conversely, anti-inflammatory foods such as leafy greens, berries, fatty fish, and turmeric can help calm the immune system. These foods are rich in antioxidants, omega-3 fatty acids, and polyphenols, which have been shown to reduce oxidative stress and promote cellular repair. Nutrient-dense diets, like the Autoimmune Protocol (AIP), focus on eliminating potential triggers and prioritizing foods that support gut health and immune regulation.

THE IMPACT OF LIFESTYLE ON AUTOIMMUNITY

Beyond diet, lifestyle factors play a crucial role in shaping immune health. Chronic stress, for example, has a profound impact on autoimmune conditions by perpetuating inflammation and suppressing the body's ability to heal. When the body is under constant stress, it produces elevated levels of cortisol, a hormone that, when dysregulated, can weaken the immune system and exacerbate autoimmune flares. Stress management techniques such as mindfulness meditation, yoga, and deep breathing exercises have been shown to reduce inflammatory markers and improve overall well-being.

Sleep is another often-overlooked factor in autoimmune health. Poor sleep quality or insufficient sleep can disrupt the body's natural repair processes and weaken immune regulation. Studies have linked sleep deprivation to increased inflammation, making it a critical focus for those managing autoimmune diseases. Establishing a consistent sleep schedule, creating a calming bedtime routine, and addressing potential sleep disorders can significantly improve health outcomes.

Physical activity, when tailored to the individual, also contributes to autoimmune management. Regular, moderate exercise helps reduce inflammation, improve circulation, and enhance mood. However, intense or excessive exercise can sometimes trigger flares in individuals with autoimmune conditions. This underscores the importance of listening to the body and choosing activities that align with one's energy levels and overall health status.

Gut Health: The Central Hub of Immunity

The gut microbiome—often referred to as the body's "second brain"—plays a pivotal role in immune function. A healthy gut microbiome fosters a balanced immune response, while dysbiosis (an imbalance in gut bacteria) can contribute to chronic inflammation and autoimmunity. Factors such as antibiotic overuse, a diet high in processed foods, and chronic stress can disrupt the microbiome, creating an environment conducive to autoimmune activity.

Restoring gut health involves both dietary and lifestyle changes. Fermented foods like sauerkraut, kimchi, and kefir introduce beneficial bacteria, while prebiotic-rich foods such as garlic, onions, and asparagus nourish these microbes. Supplements like probiotics and digestive enzymes may also be helpful, but they should be chosen carefully and under professional guidance. Additionally, reducing stress, avoiding unnecessary medications, and addressing food sensitivities are key strategies for maintaining a healthy gut environment.

Synergizing Diet and Lifestyle

The synergy between diet and lifestyle cannot be overstated in the management of autoimmunity. While dietary changes provide the building blocks for reducing inflammation and supporting immune function, lifestyle adjustments create an environment where healing can thrive. For example, a nutrient-dense diet will have limited effectiveness if chronic stress and poor sleep continue to drive inflammation. Likewise, stress management techniques may fall short if the diet is filled with inflammatory triggers.

Taking a holistic approach to health empowers individuals to take control of their autoimmune conditions. By understanding the profound influence of diet and lifestyle on the immune system, people can make informed decisions that not only alleviate symptoms but also promote long-term wellness. Although making these changes can be challenging, the rewards are undeniable—reduced inflammation, improved energy levels, and a higher quality of life await those who commit to this transformative journey.

Success Stories and Testimonials

These success stories highlight the profound impact diet and lifestyle changes can have on autoimmune diseases. Each story is unique, showcasing the versatility of AIP in managing different conditions. These testimonials are a testament to the power of determination, knowledge, and a commitment to healing through proper nutrition and lifestyle adjustments.

---

1. Sarah's Battle with Rheumatoid Arthritis: From Pain to Freedom

Sarah, a 38-year-old mother of two, had been living with rheumatoid arthritis (RA) for over a decade. She spent years on prescription medications, which provided only limited relief, and struggled with the joint pain, stiffness, and swelling that made even daily tasks feel impossible. She had been told by doctors that her condition was chronic and would only worsen over time.

In 2020, Sarah stumbled across a blog discussing AIP and its success in reversing autoimmune conditions. Skeptical but desperate for relief, she decided to give the protocol a try. The first two weeks were challenging—she faced intense detox symptoms as her body adjusted to the new way of eating. But by the end of the month, Sarah began noticing a significant reduction in her joint pain. Her morning stiffness, which used to last for hours, began to disappear. Within three months, Sarah was able to reduce her medication dosage under her doctor's supervision. By the end of six months, she was virtually pain-free, and her energy levels had returned to a level she hadn't felt in years.

Today, Sarah is thriving. She's living an active lifestyle, practicing yoga regularly, and enjoying the time with her children without the restrictions of pain. She credits AIP with transforming her life, proving that there is hope for those suffering from autoimmune diseases.

---

2. Michael's Struggle with Psoriasis: Reclaiming Skin Health

Michael, 45, had battled severe psoriasis since his twenties. His skin was covered in patches of red, inflamed lesions, and his flare-ups were often painful and uncomfortable. His condition had progressively worsened, leaving him self-conscious and socially withdrawn. He had tried numerous treatments, including topical steroids and phototherapy, but nothing provided long-term relief.

In 2021, after being recommended by a close friend, Michael decided to try the Autoimmune Protocol. Although he was initially overwhelmed by the elimination phase and the strictness of AIP, he persisted, knowing it was his last chance. The first month was tough, with his skin becoming more inflamed as his body detoxed. However, by the third month, Michael began noticing changes. His lesions started to shrink, and the redness on his scalp significantly decreased. By the end of six months, his psoriasis was nearly gone, with only a few faint patches remaining.

Now, Michael maintains an AIP diet to keep his skin clear and continues to enjoy activities like swimming and hiking without fear of flare-ups. He's able to wear short sleeves again, and his confidence has been restored.

---

3. Lisa's Healing Journey with Hashimoto's Thyroiditis: A New Lease on Life

Lisa, a 50-year-old woman, had been diagnosed with Hashimoto's thyroiditis in her late thirties. She was constantly battling fatigue, brain fog, and unexplained weight gain despite her best efforts to maintain a healthy lifestyle. Her doctors prescribed thyroid hormone replacements, but she never felt quite right. Lisa knew something deeper was at play but felt dismissed by traditional medicine.

In 2019, after hearing about AIP from a health-focused podcast, Lisa decided to give it a try. At first, the changes seemed insignificant, but by the end of the first month, Lisa noticed that her energy levels were improving. By three months, she was no longer experiencing the crushing fatigue that had once defined her daily life. Her digestion improved, her hair started to grow thicker, and her mood stabilized. After six months, Lisa's doctor ran a set of tests, revealing that her thyroid levels had significantly improved, and her antibodies had decreased.

Lisa now manages her Hashimoto's with diet, lifestyle, and stress management, and she no longer relies on medication. AIP has given her a new sense of vitality, and she is living life more fully than ever before.

---

4. Daniel's Transformation with Multiple Sclerosis: Gaining Control Over His Body

Daniel, 32, was diagnosed with multiple sclerosis (MS) at the age of 28 after experiencing numbness and tingling in his limbs, as well as fatigue. The diagnosis was life-changing, and Daniel quickly found himself dependent on multiple medications to manage the progression of his disease. The uncertainty of MS left him fearful of the future, as he witnessed his condition gradually worsen.

In 2022, after attending an MS support group, Daniel heard about the Autoimmune Protocol from another member who had seen drastic improvements in their symptoms. Daniel was determined to take control of his health and decided to follow AIP with the guidance of a nutritionist.

The first few weeks of the elimination phase were challenging, with heightened fatigue and flu-like symptoms. But after a month, Daniel started to experience fewer MS flare-ups, and his mobility improved.

Within three months, he noticed his energy levels were more stable, and his body was less prone to the sudden numbness that had previously occurred. His MRI scans also showed a reduction in lesions. Today, Daniel continues to follow AIP and is able to manage his MS without relying heavily on medication. He has regained a sense of control over his body and is optimistic about his future.

---

5. Natalie's Battle with Celiac Disease: Regaining Digestive Health

Natalie, 40, had been living with undiagnosed celiac disease for years, struggling with chronic digestive issues, bloating, and fatigue. Despite numerous tests and doctor visits, her symptoms were often misattributed to stress or other health problems. It wasn't until she sought out a functional medicine doctor in 2020 that she was properly diagnosed with celiac disease, a severe gluten intolerance that triggered autoimmune responses.

The doctor recommended that Natalie try the AIP as part of her healing process. Although she had already eliminated gluten, the strict elimination phase of AIP was an eye-opener for her. As she cut out other inflammatory foods like dairy, legumes, and nightshades, she began noticing significant improvements in her digestion. Her bloating disappeared, and she no longer suffered from painful gas or irregular bowel movements. After a few months, Natalie's energy levels skyrocketed, and her skin cleared up as well. By the end of six months, Natalie had learned to listen to her body and identify the foods that worked best for her. AIP helped her heal from the inside out, allowing her to embrace a healthy, gluten-free lifestyle without suffering from the digestive distress she had lived with for years.

These success stories reflect the transformative power of the Autoimmune Protocol in managing and reversing symptoms associated with autoimmune diseases. Each individual has found their own path to healing, demonstrating that while the journey may be difficult, the rewards of a healthier life are well worth the effort. These personal journeys are not just testimonies of healing; they are reminders that with the right knowledge, tools, and dedication, it is possible to regain control over one's health and well-being.

Content

Introduction 15
   Reclaim Your Health and Your Life 15
      Did You Know? 16
The Foundations of the Autoimmune Protocol (AIP) 18
   Origins and Evolution of AIP 18
   Core Principles of the Protocol 21
The Science Behind AIP 26
   Immune System Function and Dysfunction 26
   Gut Health: The Microbiome Connection 31
   Genetic and Environmental Influences 33
The Modified AIP Elimination Phase 37
   Foods to Eliminate 39
   Duration and Expectations 42
The Reintroduction Phase 47
   Monitoring and Identifying Food Sensitivities 51
   Meal Planning and Preparation 55
   Budget-Friendly AIP Strategies 59
Stress Management Techniques 65
   The Importance of Quality Sleep 67
   Incorporating Appropriate Physical Activity 70
   Building a Supportive Community 72
Medical Research and Evidence Supporting AIP 75
   Interpreting Research Findings 79
   Future Directions in AIP Research 81
Recipes and Meal Plans 85
   Breakfast Options 86
   Lunch and Dinner Ideas 88
   Snacks and Beverages 92

    Desserts and Treats... 96
Weekly Meal Plans and Shopping Lists.. 101
    Weekly Shopping List... 103
Conclusion.. 107
    A New Path to Healing and Wellness.. 107

Introduction

Reclaim Your Health and Your Life

In the past few decades, autoimmune diseases have become a growing concern worldwide. Affecting millions of people across different ages, backgrounds, and health profiles, these conditions have skyrocketed in prevalence. According to the American Autoimmune Related Diseases Association (AARDA), approximately **50 million Americans** suffer from an autoimmune disease, making them one of the leading causes of chronic illness. But here's the reality: **autoimmune diseases are not simply genetic**. In fact, research has shown that **environmental factors**—such as diet, stress, and toxins—play a critical role in triggering or exacerbating these conditions. The good news is that **diet and lifestyle changes can have a profound impact on managing and even reversing autoimmune diseases**.

If you're reading this book, it's likely that you, or someone you care about, has been affected by an autoimmune disorder. You might be tired of trying one medication after another, experiencing side effects, or feeling frustrated that conventional treatments only address symptoms, not the root cause of the disease. You may have been told that autoimmune conditions are chronic, progressive, and incurable—but what if there was another way?

The Autoimmune Protocol (AIP) offers a powerful alternative, rooted in scientific research and years of clinical practice, designed to help individuals address the underlying causes of autoimmune disease. This protocol is not just another fad diet or trendy wellness recommendation. It is a **scientifically grounded, step-by-step approach** to **healing**—by addressing the body's root causes of inflammation and restoring balance to the immune system through food and lifestyle changes.

But why does this approach work? The answer lies in the **gut-immune connection**. Studies have shown that **over 70% of the immune system** resides in the gut, which is responsible for regulating inflammation and immune responses. When the gut becomes damaged or imbalanced, it can trigger an autoimmune response—attacking the body's own tissues and organs. By healing the gut and eliminating foods that fuel this immune dysfunction, the body has a chance to restore normal immune function and reduce chronic inflammation.

In this book, you will learn how the Autoimmune Protocol works, why it's effective, and how you can implement it to take control of your health. With the proven benefits of this protocol—such as improved energy, better digestion, reduced inflammation, and symptom relief—more and more people are embracing it as a way to **reverse autoimmune conditions**, regain their health, and live vibrant, fulfilling lives.

Did You Know?

- An estimated **1 in 9 women** will develop an autoimmune disease in their lifetime. Some of the most common conditions include Hashimoto's thyroiditis, rheumatoid arthritis, and lupus.
- Studies have shown that **up to 80% of people with autoimmune conditions experience symptoms related to gut health**, such as bloating, indigestion, and food sensitivities.
- **Dietary changes**—including the elimination of certain inflammatory foods—have been shown to significantly improve symptoms in individuals with autoimmune diseases, with many reporting relief within just a few weeks of following the protocol.

If you've been living with the frustration of autoimmune disease, wondering if there's hope for better health, this book will show you that there is. Through the principles of the Autoimmune Protocol, you will discover how to take control of your body's healing process, with a clear roadmap for diet, lifestyle changes, and ongoing support.

This is more than just a book about managing autoimmune disease. It's a **guide to reclaiming your health, your vitality, and your future**. Whether you're dealing with an autoimmune condition yourself or seeking to prevent one, *The Autoimmune Protocol* offers the knowledge, tools, and inspiration you need to transform your health and live a life free from the constraints of chronic illness.

The Foundations of the Autoimmune Protocol (AIP)

Origins and Evolution of AIP

The Autoimmune Protocol (AIP) has emerged as a transformative approach to managing autoimmune diseases, rooted in addressing the root causes of immune dysfunction through targeted dietary and lifestyle interventions.

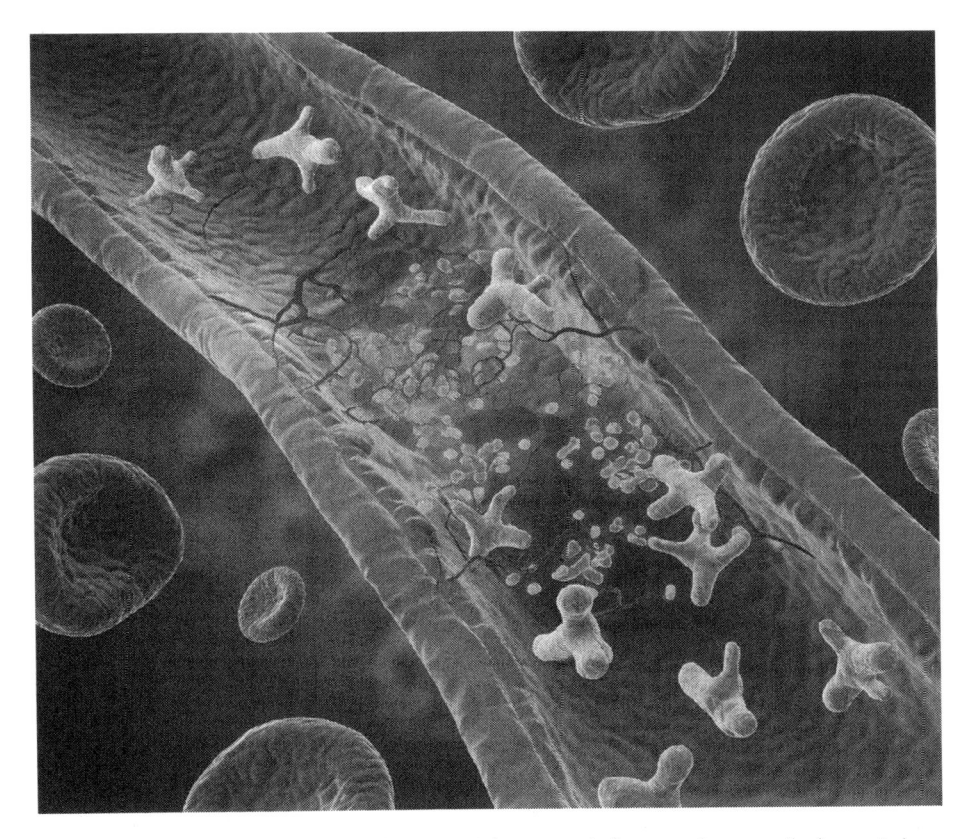

To fully appreciate its significance, it's essential to understand the origins, evolution, and scientific principles that form the backbone of this innovative protocol.

The development of the Autoimmune Protocol is credited to the pioneering efforts of clinicians, researchers, and nutrition experts who recognized the limitations of conventional medical treatments for autoimmune diseases. Traditional approaches primarily focus on suppressing immune activity through medications such as corticosteroids, biologics, or immunosuppressants. While these treatments often provide symptom relief, they do little to address the underlying causes of autoimmunity and may come with significant side effects.

The AIP began as an alternative framework, grounded in functional and integrative medicine principles. This approach views the body as an interconnected system, emphasizing the role of inflammation, gut health, and environmental triggers in autoimmune disease development. Early proponents of AIP, such as Dr. Sarah Ballantyne, also known as "The Paleo Mom," and other thought leaders in the field, sought to create a holistic, evidence-based strategy to restore immune balance by modifying diet and lifestyle.

Building on the Paleo Diet Foundation

The roots of the Autoimmune Protocol lie in the Paleo Diet, a nutritional approach based on the dietary habits of our Paleolithic ancestors. The Paleo Diet emphasizes whole, unprocessed foods such as vegetables, fruits, lean meats, fish, nuts, and seeds while eliminating grains, legumes, dairy, and processed foods. Early adopters of the Paleo Diet reported improvements in autoimmune symptoms, sparking interest in its potential as a therapeutic intervention for immune dysfunction.

However, researchers and practitioners soon recognized that additional refinements were necessary to cater specifically to individuals with autoimmune diseases. Certain foods deemed acceptable in the standard Paleo Diet, such as nuts, seeds, eggs, and nightshade vegetables (e.g., tomatoes, peppers, and eggplants), were found to trigger immune responses in some individuals with autoimmune conditions. These observations led to the development of the Autoimmune Protocol, a more restrictive and targeted dietary framework designed to eliminate potential triggers and promote healing.

Since its inception, the Autoimmune Protocol has evolved through ongoing research and clinical practice. The initial focus was on dietary modifications, specifically the elimination of foods known to promote inflammation, irritate the gut lining, or overstimulate the immune system. Over time, practitioners recognized the importance of reintroducing foods systematically to identify individual sensitivities and create a sustainable, personalized diet.

Beyond diet, the AIP has expanded to encompass lifestyle factors that profoundly influence immune health. Stress management, quality sleep, physical activity, and social support are now integral components of the protocol. This holistic approach acknowledges that autoimmune diseases are multifactorial and require a comprehensive strategy to address the physical, emotional, and environmental aspects of health.

As awareness of the Autoimmune Protocol has grown, so too has the body of scientific evidence supporting its efficacy. Clinical studies have demonstrated that AIP can significantly reduce symptoms and improve quality of life for individuals with autoimmune diseases such as inflammatory bowel disease, Hashimoto's thyroiditis, and rheumatoid arthritis. These findings have bolstered the credibility of AIP within the medical and scientific communities, leading to increased adoption by practitioners and patients alike.

The success of AIP has also been amplified by personal testimonials and case studies shared through books, blogs, and social media platforms. These stories of transformative healing have inspired countless individuals to explore AIP as a viable solution for managing their autoimmune conditions, further cementing its place as a cornerstone of functional medicine.

The Autoimmune Protocol continues to evolve as research sheds new light on the complex interplay between diet, lifestyle, and immune health. Emerging studies on the gut microbiome, epigenetics, and the impact of environmental toxins are likely to inform future iterations of the protocol. Additionally, the development of modified versions of AIP, such as the 2024 "Modified AIP," reflects the need for adaptability and inclusivity in addressing the diverse needs of individuals with autoimmune diseases.

As we move forward, the AIP remains a beacon of hope for those seeking to take control of their health through natural and sustainable means. By understanding its origins and embracing its evolution, individuals can embark on a journey of healing that empowers them to live vibrant, fulfilling lives despite the challenges of autoimmunity.

Core Principles of the Protocol

Distinguishing AIP from Other Dietary Approaches

The Autoimmune Protocol (AIP) is not merely a diet but a comprehensive lifestyle framework designed to address the underlying drivers of autoimmune disease. While it shares similarities with other dietary approaches, such as the Paleo Diet or anti-inflammatory diets, it stands out due to its targeted focus on immune system regulation, gut health, and personalized healing. Understanding these core principles and how they differ from other methods provides clarity on why AIP is uniquely effective for managing autoimmune conditions.

1. Prioritizing Elimination and Reintroduction

The cornerstone of the AIP is its structured elimination and reintroduction process, which goes beyond the simple removal of harmful foods. The protocol begins with a highly restrictive phase, eliminating potential inflammatory triggers such as:

- Gluten, dairy, grains, and legumes
- Nightshade vegetables (e.g., tomatoes, peppers, eggplants, potatoes)
- Seeds, nuts, and seed-based oils
- Eggs, caffeine, alcohol, and all processed or refined foods

The goal is to reduce immune system activation and inflammation by removing foods that may irritate the gut lining, disrupt the microbiome, or stimulate an overactive immune response. Once symptoms stabilize and the individual experiences improvement, foods are reintroduced systematically and slowly to identify specific sensitivities.

This targeted process distinguishes AIP from generalized diets that focus solely on elimination without reintroducing foods in a methodical way. It allows for personalized adjustments that cater to each individual's unique triggers, fostering long-term sustainability.

2. Focus on Gut Health

Unlike many other diets, the AIP emphasizes the critical role of gut health in autoimmune disease management. Scientific studies have shown that a compromised gut barrier, often referred to as "leaky gut," is a common factor in autoimmunity. When the gut lining is damaged, harmful substances such as toxins, undigested food particles, and pathogens can leak into the bloodstream, triggering an immune response.

The AIP specifically incorporates foods and strategies that promote gut healing, such as:

- **Bone broth:** Rich in collagen and amino acids that support gut lining repair
- **Fermented foods:** Like sauerkraut and kimchi, which introduce beneficial probiotics to restore microbiome balance
- **Prebiotic-rich vegetables:** Such as asparagus and garlic, to nourish good gut bacteria
- **Nutrient-dense options:** Like organ meats and shellfish, which provide essential vitamins and minerals

This gut-centered approach is far more nuanced than general anti-inflammatory diets, making AIP particularly suited for those with autoimmune conditions.

3. Nutrient Density Above All Else

The AIP prioritizes nutrient density to ensure the body receives the building blocks it needs for repair and immune regulation. Unlike some restrictive diets that can lead to nutrient deficiencies, the AIP focuses on including a wide variety of foods rich in vitamins, minerals, and antioxidants. Examples of nutrient-dense foods encouraged on the protocol include:

- Leafy greens such as kale, spinach, and Swiss chard
- Wild-caught fish like salmon and mackerel, high in omega-3 fatty acids
- Root vegetables like sweet potatoes and parsnips, providing complex carbohydrates
- Organ meats like liver, packed with essential nutrients like vitamin A and iron

This focus sets the AIP apart from other dietary approaches that may limit certain food groups without accounting for nutritional balance.

4. A Holistic Lifestyle Framework

While diet is a central component of the AIP, it is not the sole focus. The protocol integrates lifestyle modifications to create a holistic healing environment. This includes:

- **Stress management:** Chronic stress exacerbates inflammation and immune dysregulation. Practices like mindfulness, yoga, and journaling are integral to AIP.
- **Sleep optimization:** Prioritizing 7-9 hours of restorative sleep to support the body's natural repair processes.
- **Gentle physical activity:** Encouraging movement such as walking, yoga, or swimming, while avoiding high-intensity exercises that may trigger flares.
- **Toxin reduction:** Limiting exposure to environmental toxins through natural cleaning products, organic foods, and clean water sources.

This comprehensive focus distinguishes AIP from traditional diets that often neglect the role of stress, sleep, and environmental factors in immune health.

5. Personalization and Flexibility

Unlike rigid one-size-fits-all dietary plans, the AIP is inherently adaptable to individual needs. After the elimination and reintroduction phases, the protocol allows individuals to tailor their diet based on their unique triggers, sensitivities, and lifestyle preferences. This personalized approach makes the AIP sustainable in the long term, empowering individuals to maintain their health without feeling overly restricted.

By contrast, other dietary approaches often lack this level of customization, leading to frustration or failure when specific needs are not addressed.

6. Evidence-Based Framework

The AIP is grounded in scientific research and clinical evidence, which adds to its credibility and effectiveness. Studies have demonstrated significant improvements in autoimmune conditions, such as reduced inflammatory markers, symptom relief, and improved quality of life, for individuals following the AIP. Its emphasis on scientific validation distinguishes it from fad diets or anecdotal wellness trends.

How AIP Stands Out

While other diets, such as the Mediterranean, ketogenic, or low-FODMAP diets, offer benefits, they are not specifically tailored to the unique challenges of autoimmune diseases. The AIP stands out by addressing:

- The root causes of immune dysfunction
- The connection between diet, gut health, and systemic inflammation
- The holistic integration of lifestyle factors

Through its comprehensive approach, the AIP has established itself as a transformative protocol for managing autoimmune diseases and achieving long-term wellness. By understanding and embracing these core principles, individuals with autoimmune conditions can embark on a path to healing that is rooted in science, personalization, and sustainable health practices.

The Science Behind AIP

Immune System Function and Dysfunction

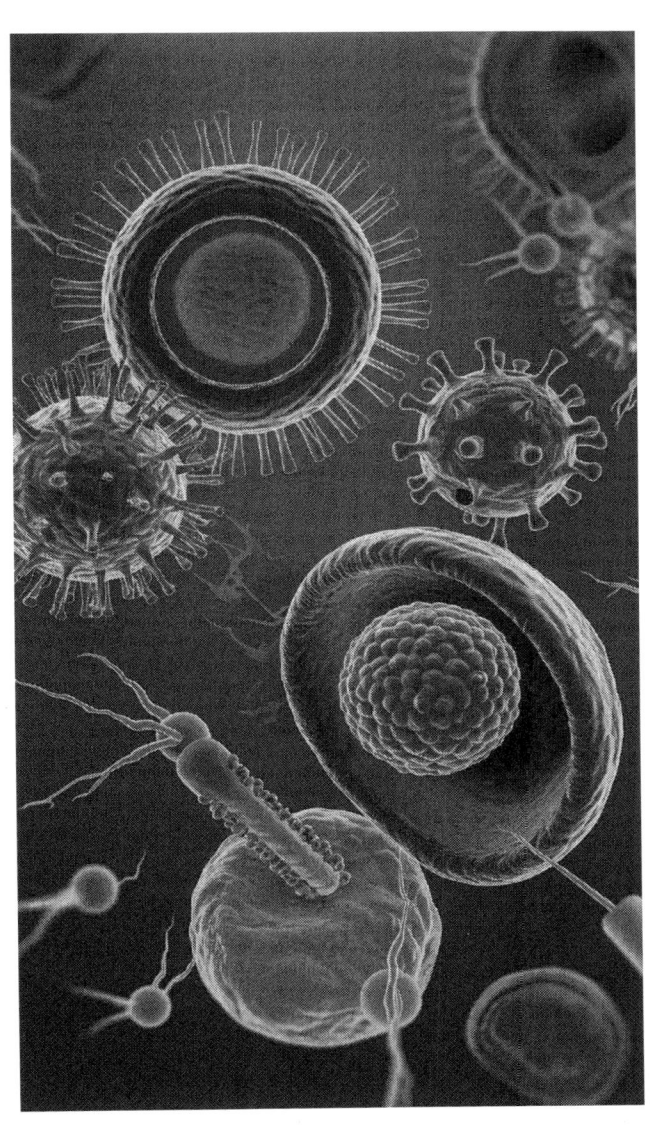

The immune system is a complex network of cells, tissues, and organs designed to protect the body from harmful invaders such as bacteria, viruses, and toxins. It operates with remarkable precision, identifying and eliminating threats while distinguishing them from the body's own healthy cells. However, in individuals with autoimmune diseases, this system malfunctions, attacking healthy tissues and organs as though they were foreign invaders. Understanding the science behind this dysfunction is essential to appreciating the role of the Autoimmune Protocol (AIP) in restoring balance and mitigating immune-related damage.

The Basics of Immune System Function

The immune system has two primary components:

1. **Innate Immunity:** The first line of defense, providing nonspecific protection through physical barriers (e.g., skin, mucous membranes) and immune cells like macrophages and neutrophils.
2. **Adaptive Immunity:** A more specialized system involving T cells and B cells that target specific pathogens. This system has memory, allowing the body to respond more efficiently to previously encountered threats.

When functioning properly, the immune system maintains a state of tolerance, ensuring it does not react against the body's own tissues. This balance is regulated by mechanisms such as regulatory T cells (Tregs), which suppress overactive immune responses.

Dysfunction in Autoimmune Diseases

In autoimmune diseases, this balance is disrupted, leading to a state where the immune system mistakenly identifies the body's own tissues as threats. This process is driven by several key factors:

1. **Molecular Mimicry:** Sometimes, pathogens share structural similarities with human tissues. When the immune system attacks the pathogen, it may inadvertently target the body's own cells. For example, this mechanism is thought to contribute to conditions like rheumatoid arthritis and multiple sclerosis.

2. **Loss of Immune Tolerance**: Regulatory T cells fail to suppress overactive immune responses, allowing self-reactive immune cells to attack healthy tissues.
3. **Genetic Susceptibility**: Certain genetic variations, such as those in the HLA (human leukocyte antigen) genes, increase the likelihood of developing autoimmune diseases by affecting how the immune system recognizes self and non-self.
4. **Environmental Triggers**: Factors such as infections, toxins, stress, and dietary antigens can activate the immune system in susceptible individuals, contributing to the onset or exacerbation of autoimmune diseases.

The result is chronic inflammation, tissue damage, and the progression of autoimmune conditions, such as lupus, Hashimoto's thyroiditis, or psoriasis.

The Role of AIP in Immune Regulation

The Autoimmune Protocol targets immune dysfunction by addressing key drivers of autoimmunity. Through its elimination phase, the AIP removes dietary and environmental triggers that may overstimulate the immune system or compromise gut health. By focusing on nutrient-dense, anti-inflammatory foods, the protocol supports the immune system in restoring tolerance and reducing unnecessary immune activation.

Chronic Inflammation and Its Role in Autoimmunity

Inflammation is a natural and essential response of the immune system to injury or infection. It involves the release of signaling molecules, such as cytokines, that recruit immune cells to the affected area to combat pathogens or facilitate tissue repair. However, when inflammation becomes chronic, it transitions from a protective mechanism to a destructive process, fueling the development and progression of autoimmune diseases.

Chronic inflammation occurs when the immune system remains persistently activated, even in the absence of an ongoing threat. This state can arise due to unresolved infections, exposure to environmental toxins, or sustained dietary insults. Over time, chronic inflammation damages tissues and organs, disrupting their function and leading to symptoms such as pain, fatigue, and organ dysfunction.

Key drivers of chronic inflammation include:

1. **Leaky Gut Syndrome**: A compromised intestinal barrier allows harmful substances, such as undigested food particles and bacterial toxins, to enter the bloodstream. This triggers an immune response, perpetuating systemic inflammation.
2. **Pro-Inflammatory Diets**: Diets high in refined sugars, trans fats, processed foods, and artificial additives contribute to the production of inflammatory cytokines. Certain foods, like gluten and dairy, may also act as triggers in susceptible individuals.
3. **Oxidative Stress**: An imbalance between free radicals and antioxidants in the body leads to cellular damage and inflammation.
4. **Environmental Exposures**: Pollutants, heavy metals, and chronic stress can activate inflammatory pathways.

In autoimmune diseases, chronic inflammation becomes a self-perpetuating cycle. The immune system's attack on healthy tissues causes further tissue damage, releasing cellular debris that the immune system perceives as a threat. This creates a feedback loop, intensifying inflammation and accelerating the disease process.

For example:

- In **rheumatoid arthritis**, chronic inflammation damages joints, leading to pain, swelling, and reduced mobility.

- In **Hashimoto's thyroiditis**, inflammation in the thyroid gland impairs its ability to produce hormones, causing hypothyroidism.
- In **lupus**, systemic inflammation affects multiple organs, leading to widespread symptoms.

How AIP Mitigates Chronic Inflammation

The Autoimmune Protocol is specifically designed to break the cycle of chronic inflammation through dietary and lifestyle interventions:

1. **Elimination of Inflammatory Foods:** By removing foods known to trigger immune responses, such as gluten, dairy, and nightshades, the AIP reduces the inflammatory burden on the body.
2. **Gut Healing:** Incorporating gut-supportive foods, like bone broth and fermented vegetables, repairs the intestinal barrier, preventing the entry of inflammatory substances into the bloodstream.
3. **Antioxidant-Rich Diet:** Foods rich in antioxidants, such as leafy greens and berries, neutralize free radicals, reducing oxidative stress and inflammation.
4. **Stress Reduction:** Mindfulness practices and stress management techniques lower cortisol levels, a hormone that, when elevated chronically, can exacerbate inflammation.
5. **Holistic Lifestyle Changes:** Adequate sleep, gentle exercise, and toxin reduction further support the body's natural anti-inflammatory mechanisms.

By addressing immune dysfunction and chronic inflammation at their roots, the Autoimmune Protocol offers a pathway to symptom relief and long-term healing. It empowers individuals to take control of their health, reduce the burden of autoimmune disease, and restore vitality through natural, evidence-based strategies. Through the lens of science, AIP provides hope for reversing the destructive cycle of autoimmunity and reclaiming wellness.

Gut Health: The Microbiome Connection

The gut is often referred to as the "second brain" due to its profound impact on overall health, particularly its connection to the immune system. The trillions of microorganisms that reside in the gastrointestinal tract, collectively known as the gut microbiome, play a pivotal role in maintaining immune balance, supporting digestion, and protecting against pathogens. When the microbiome is disrupted, it can become a significant driver of autoimmune disease, making it a critical focus of the Autoimmune Protocol (AIP).

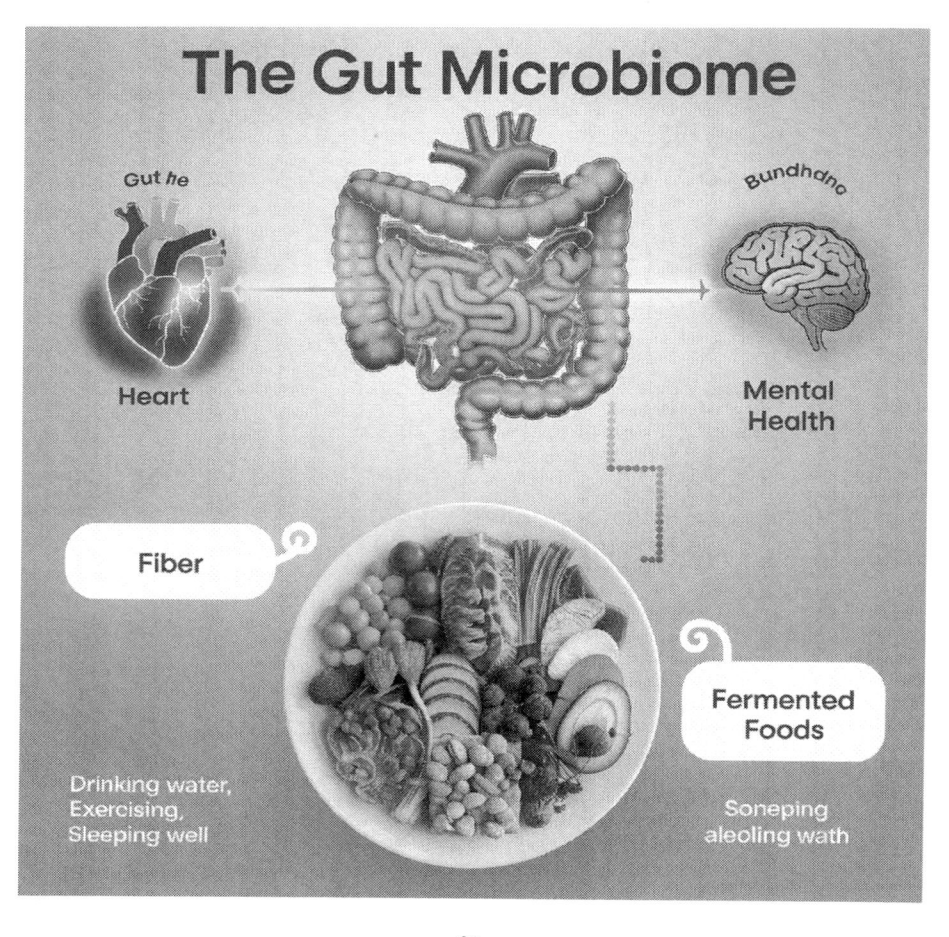

The Role of the Gut Microbiome in Immune Regulation

Approximately 70% of the immune system is housed in the gut, highlighting the intimate connection between gut health and immune function. The microbiome has several key roles:

1. **Maintaining the Intestinal Barrier**: Beneficial gut bacteria strengthen the lining of the intestines, preventing harmful substances like toxins, pathogens, and undigested food particles from entering the bloodstream.
2. **Modulating Immune Responses**: The microbiome educates the immune system, teaching it to differentiate between harmful invaders and the body's own tissues. Dysbiosis, an imbalance in gut bacteria, can lead to inappropriate immune activation and inflammation.
3. **Producing Short-Chain Fatty Acids (SCFAs)**: These anti-inflammatory compounds, produced by gut bacteria during the fermentation of dietary fiber, support immune health and help maintain the integrity of the gut lining.

One of the most critical links between gut health and autoimmune disease is leaky gut syndrome, also known as increased intestinal permeability. In this condition, the tight junctions that seal the gut lining become compromised, allowing harmful substances to pass into the bloodstream.

This triggers a cascade of immune responses:

- The immune system identifies these substances as threats and mounts an inflammatory response.
- Over time, this chronic inflammation can lead to immune system dysregulation and the development of autoimmune diseases.

Leaky gut is frequently observed in autoimmune conditions such as celiac disease, Crohn's disease, and rheumatoid arthritis. Addressing gut health through the AIP can help repair the gut lining, restore microbiome balance, and reduce systemic inflammation.

Restoring Gut Health with AIP

The Autoimmune Protocol emphasizes gut health as a cornerstone of healing. Key strategies include:

1. **Eliminating Gut Irritants**: Foods like gluten, dairy, and refined sugars are removed because they can contribute to leaky gut and dysbiosis.
2. **Incorporating Gut-Healing Foods**:
    - **Bone Broth**: Rich in collagen and amino acids, it supports gut lining repair.
    - **Fermented Foods**: Such as sauerkraut and kimchi, which promote a diverse and balanced microbiome.
    - **Prebiotic Foods**: Like garlic and asparagus, which nourish beneficial gut bacteria.
3. **Avoiding Environmental Toxins**: Reducing exposure to pesticides, heavy metals, and artificial additives helps minimize gut inflammation.
4. **Managing Stress**: Chronic stress can disrupt the gut-brain axis, compromising both gut health and immune function.

By focusing on these principles, the AIP helps rebuild the gut microbiome, strengthen the intestinal barrier, and restore immune balance.

Genetic and Environmental Influences

Autoimmune diseases arise from a complex interplay of genetic predispositions and environmental factors. While genetics create the blueprint, environmental triggers often determine whether an autoimmune condition develops and how it progresses. Understanding these influences is essential for tailoring the AIP to individual needs.

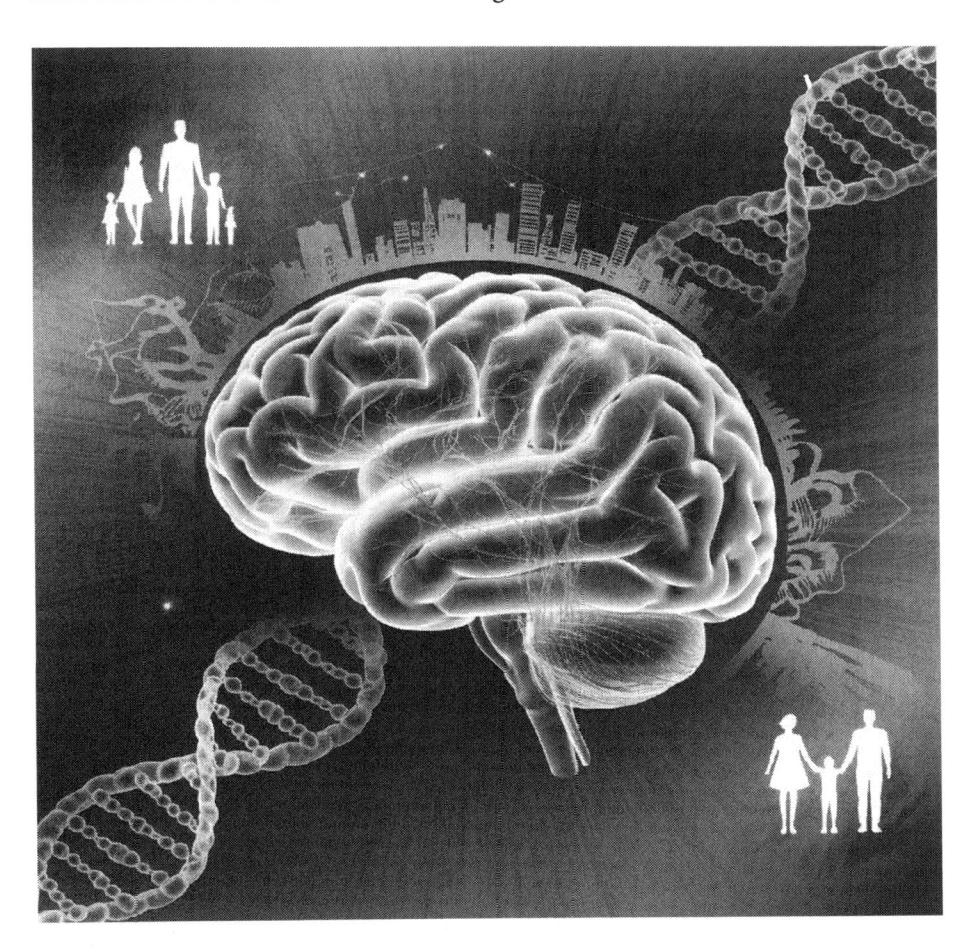

Genetic Susceptibility

Certain genetic variations, particularly those in the HLA (human leukocyte antigen) genes, increase the likelihood of autoimmune disease. The HLA complex plays a critical role in presenting antigens to immune cells, and mutations in these genes can impair the immune system's ability to distinguish between self and non-self.

However, genetics alone do not guarantee the development of autoimmunity. Studies suggest that genetics account for only 30% of the risk, with the remaining 70% attributed to environmental and lifestyle factors.

Environmental Triggers

Environmental factors act as the "on switch" for autoimmune diseases in genetically susceptible individuals. Key triggers include:

1. **Diet**: Pro-inflammatory diets high in processed foods, refined sugars, and unhealthy fats contribute to systemic inflammation and immune dysregulation.
2. **Infections**: Viral or bacterial infections can activate the immune system and trigger molecular mimicry, where the immune system attacks healthy tissues resembling the pathogen.
3. **Toxins**: Exposure to heavy metals, pesticides, and other environmental toxins can disrupt immune function and damage tissues.
4. **Stress**: Chronic stress elevates cortisol levels, which can weaken the immune system and exacerbate inflammation.
5. **Gut Dysbiosis**: Imbalances in gut bacteria, often caused by antibiotic overuse, poor diet, or stress, are a significant driver of autoimmunity.

Epigenetics: The Link Between Genes and Environment

Epigenetics refers to changes in gene expression caused by environmental factors, rather than alterations in the genetic code itself. For example:

- A pro-inflammatory diet or chronic stress can "turn on" genes associated with autoimmunity, increasing disease risk.

- Conversely, adopting an anti-inflammatory lifestyle through AIP can "turn off" these genes, reducing symptoms and promoting healing.

Addressing Genetic and Environmental Factors Through AIP

The Autoimmune Protocol provides a comprehensive approach to mitigating genetic and environmental risks:

- **Dietary Adjustments:** Removing pro-inflammatory foods and incorporating nutrient-dense options reduces genetic expression of inflammatory markers.
- **Lifestyle Changes:** Stress management, toxin reduction, and improved sleep quality mitigate environmental triggers.
- **Personalized Approach:** Recognizing individual genetic and environmental influences allows for tailored adjustments, ensuring the protocol meets specific needs.

By addressing both genetic and environmental factors, the AIP empowers individuals to take control of their health, minimize disease triggers, and promote long-term well-being.

The Modified AIP Elimination Phase

The Autoimmune Protocol (AIP) is a dynamic dietary framework designed to address and reverse autoimmune conditions by systematically eliminating inflammatory and potentially harmful foods. In 2024, the protocol underwent a significant update, introducing a modified approach to the elimination phase. This chapter provides an in-depth guide to understanding and implementing the updated elimination phase for optimal results.

Introduction to Modified AIP (2024 Update)

The modified AIP reflects the latest advancements in nutrition science and immunology, ensuring a more personalized and accessible approach to managing autoimmune diseases. While the core principles remain intact, the updated protocol introduces flexibility and refinements based on emerging research and individual needs.

Key highlights of the 2024 update include:

- **Enhanced Personalization**: Recognizing bio-individuality, the protocol allows adjustments for specific conditions and dietary tolerances.
- **Focus on Nutritional Sufficiency**: Emphasizing a broader range of nutrient-dense foods to prevent deficiencies and support healing.
- **Incorporation of New Research**: Integrating findings on gut health, immune regulation, and the microbiome to refine food choices and lifestyle recommendations.

The modified AIP elimination phase remains a cornerstone of the protocol, providing a structured approach to identify food triggers, reduce inflammation, and reset the immune system.

Rationale and Development

The elimination phase is not merely about removing certain foods; it is a strategic process rooted in scientific understanding of how diet impacts autoimmune conditions.

- **Addressing Inflammatory Triggers:** Certain foods contain compounds like gluten, lectins, or processed oils, which can irritate the gut lining, disrupt the microbiome, and fuel systemic inflammation. Removing these foods allows the body to heal.
- **Resetting the Immune System:** Chronic exposure to dietary triggers can confuse the immune system, causing it to attack healthy tissues. The elimination phase helps calm this hyperactivity.
- **Restoring Gut Health:** By removing irritants, the gut lining has the opportunity to repair itself, strengthening the intestinal barrier and reducing leaky gut.
- **Identifying Food Sensitivities:** Through elimination and reintroduction, individuals can pinpoint specific foods that exacerbate symptoms, enabling a tailored dietary approach.

The development of the modified AIP elimination phase also took into account feedback from practitioners and patients, ensuring it is both effective and sustainable for a diverse population.

Foods to Eliminate

The elimination phase involves temporarily removing foods that are known or suspected to contribute to inflammation, immune dysregulation, or gut irritation. The 2024 update refines this list to include:

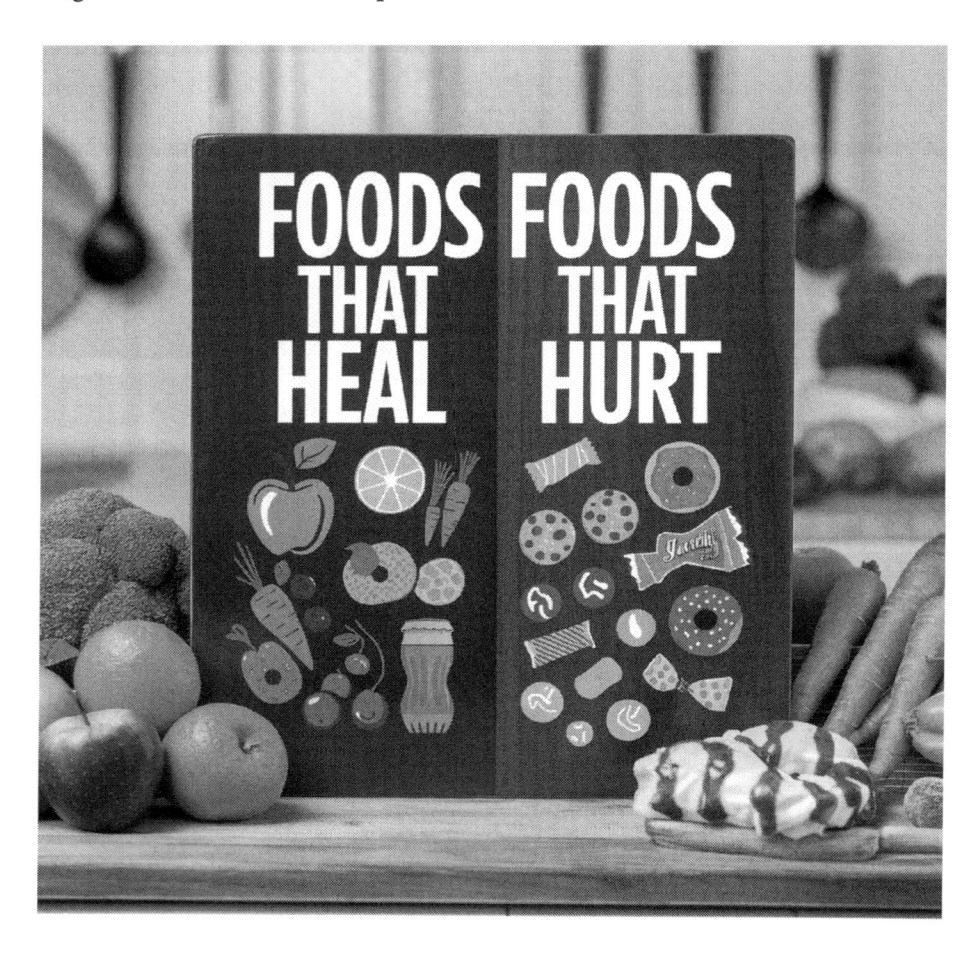

1. **Grains:**
    - Gluten-containing grains (wheat, barley, rye)
    - Gluten-free grains (rice, corn, oats, quinoa)
      Rationale: Grains contain lectins and phytates that can

irritate the gut lining and exacerbate autoimmune symptoms.

2. **Legumes:**
   - Beans, lentils, peanuts, soy products
     Rationale: Legumes are rich in lectins and can be difficult to digest, leading to inflammation in susceptible individuals.

3. **Dairy:**
   - Milk, cheese, yogurt, butter (including clarified butter in this phase)
     Rationale: Dairy proteins, such as casein, can trigger immune responses, and lactose can contribute to gut dysbiosis.

4. **Processed Foods:**
   - Packaged snacks, artificial additives, preservatives, and refined sugars
     Rationale: These foods are devoid of nutrients and can drive inflammation and oxidative stress.

5. **Refined and Industrial Oils:**
   - Canola, soybean, corn, and other vegetable oils
     Rationale: High in omega-6 fatty acids, these oils promote inflammation.

6. **Nuts and Seeds:**
   - Almonds, walnuts, sunflower seeds, sesame seeds, and nut-based flours or butters
     Rationale: Though nutrient-dense, nuts and seeds can be difficult to digest and may irritate the gut in sensitive individuals.

7. **Nightshades:**
   - Tomatoes, peppers (including chili and bell peppers), eggplants, white potatoes
     Rationale: Nightshades contain alkaloids, which can

stimulate an immune response and aggravate inflammation in some people.

8. **Eggs:**
   - Both egg whites and yolks
   Rationale: Egg whites contain proteins that can act as antigens, while the yolks can be inflammatory for certain individuals.

9. **Caffeine and Alcohol:**
   - Coffee, tea, energy drinks, wine, beer, spirits
   Rationale: These substances can irritate the gut lining, disrupt sleep, and exacerbate autoimmune symptoms.

10. **Sweeteners and Sugars:**

- Refined sugars, artificial sweeteners, and natural sweeteners like honey (in the initial phase)
Rationale: Excessive sugar consumption contributes to systemic inflammation and disrupts the microbiome.

Additional Considerations

The modified AIP recognizes that some foods may be well-tolerated by certain individuals, even if they are typically restricted. Working with a healthcare professional or an AIP-experienced practitioner can help determine whether specific modifications are appropriate.

Moreover, the elimination phase is designed to be temporary. It typically lasts 30–90 days, depending on the severity of symptoms and individual progress. The goal is to heal the body and gather insights for long-term dietary adjustments.

By adhering to the updated elimination guidelines, individuals can create a strong foundation for healing, addressing the root causes of their autoimmune conditions and setting the stage for sustained recovery.

Duration and Expectations

The elimination phase of the Autoimmune Protocol (AIP) is a temporary yet transformative step in healing autoimmune conditions. Its purpose is to reset the body, reduce inflammation, and identify dietary triggers through systematic food elimination and reintroduction.

How Long Should the Elimination Phase Last?

The duration of the elimination phase is typically **30 to 90 days**, though this may vary based on individual progress and the severity of autoimmune symptoms.

- **Mild Symptoms:** Individuals with mild or newly diagnosed autoimmune conditions may notice improvements within 4–6 weeks.
- **Severe or Longstanding Conditions:** For those with more advanced or chronic issues, the elimination phase may extend to 90 days or more.

The ultimate goal is to reach a point where symptoms stabilize or improve significantly. This period is essential to allow the body to heal, restore the gut lining, and reduce systemic inflammation. Once noticeable progress is achieved, the reintroduction phase can begin to identify which foods can be safely reintroduced without triggering symptoms.

What to Expect During the Elimination Phase

1. **Early Adjustments:**
    - The first 1–2 weeks may feel challenging as your body adjusts to the removal of common allergens and inflammatory foods. You might experience withdrawal symptoms, such as fatigue, irritability, or cravings, particularly for sugar and caffeine.

- These symptoms are temporary and are often a sign that your body is detoxifying.
2. **Symptom Improvement:**
    - By weeks 3–4, many individuals begin to notice reduced inflammation, better digestion, improved energy levels, and fewer autoimmune flare-ups.
    - Symptoms such as joint pain, brain fog, and fatigue often decrease as the body starts to heal.
3. **Healing Plateaus:**
    - It's normal to experience plateaus where progress slows or stalls. These periods are an opportunity to reassess factors like sleep, stress management, and adherence to the protocol.
4. **Long-Term Awareness:**
    - By the end of the elimination phase, you will have a clearer understanding of how food impacts your health. This knowledge will guide your reintroduction process and inform long-term dietary choices.

Patience is key during this phase, as the timeline for healing varies widely based on individual circumstances.

Common Challenges and Solutions

Embarking on the AIP elimination phase can be transformative but also presents unique challenges. Awareness and preparation can help overcome these obstacles and ensure success.

1. Difficulty Adjusting to New Foods

Challenge: Transitioning from a standard diet to AIP can feel restrictive, with unfamiliar foods and limited options.
Solution:

- Focus on abundance rather than restriction by exploring the wide range of nutrient-dense AIP-friendly foods.
- Experiment with AIP-approved recipes and flavor profiles to make meals enjoyable and satisfying.
- Meal planning and batch cooking can reduce stress and ensure you always have compliant options on hand.

2. Managing Cravings

Challenge: Cravings for eliminated foods, especially sugar, caffeine, and processed snacks, are common in the early days of the protocol.
Solution:

- Replace cravings with nutrient-dense snacks like AIP-friendly smoothies, avocado with sea salt, or roasted vegetables.
- Stay hydrated and include healthy fats in your meals to promote satiety and reduce sugar cravings.
- Use mindfulness techniques like deep breathing or journaling to address emotional triggers for cravings.

3. Social and Cultural Challenges

Challenge: Social gatherings, dining out, and cultural traditions can be difficult to navigate while following AIP.
Solution:

- Communicate your dietary needs to friends and family in advance, and consider bringing your own AIP-compliant dishes to gatherings.
- Research restaurant menus ahead of time or call to ask about ingredient flexibility.
- Embrace the opportunity to educate others about your journey and the importance of prioritizing your health.

4. Financial and Time Constraints

Challenge: Sourcing organic, grass-fed, and AIP-compliant foods can feel expensive or time-consuming.
Solution:

- Prioritize the most impactful changes, such as switching to organic produce for the "Dirty Dozen" and focusing on gut-healing staples like bone broth and fermented vegetables.
- Shop in bulk, freeze leftovers, and utilize farmers' markets or online sources for cost-effective options.
- Plan meals ahead of time to reduce food waste and time spent deciding what to eat.

5. Emotional and Psychological Impact

Challenge: Adhering to a strict dietary protocol can sometimes feel isolating or overwhelming, especially in the face of slow progress.
Solution:

- Focus on the "why" behind your efforts, reminding yourself of your long-term health goals.
- Join AIP support groups or online communities for encouragement, recipe ideas, and shared experiences.
- Practice self-care beyond diet, such as yoga, meditation, or hobbies that bring joy and reduce stress.

6. Healing Crisis or Flare-Ups

Challenge: Some individuals experience temporary symptom flare-ups as the body detoxifies and adjusts.
Solution:

- Understand that this is part of the healing process for many and does not indicate failure.
- Stay consistent with the protocol while ensuring proper hydration, rest, and stress reduction.
- Consult a healthcare provider if symptoms persist or worsen to rule out underlying issues.

The Reintroduction Phase

The reintroduction phase of the Autoimmune Protocol (AIP) is a critical step in identifying personal food triggers and expanding your diet while maintaining the healing achieved during the elimination phase. This chapter explores the purpose of reintroduction, its importance, and a systematic process to help individuals reintroduce foods safely and effectively.

Purpose and Importance of Reintroduction

While the elimination phase focuses on reducing inflammation and allowing the body to heal, the reintroduction phase is essential for long-term dietary sustainability and personalization. It serves several key purposes:

1. **Identifying Food Triggers:**
   - Autoimmune responses and inflammatory symptoms often stem from specific food sensitivities or intolerances. The reintroduction phase helps pinpoint these triggers by reintroducing one food at a time and observing the body's reaction.
2. **Expanding Dietary Diversity:**
   - A diverse diet is essential for gut health, nutrient intake, and maintaining a robust microbiome. Reintroduction allows individuals to safely incorporate a wider variety of nutrient-dense foods into their meals.
3. **Reducing Dietary Restrictions:**
   - Overly restrictive diets can lead to nutrient deficiencies, social isolation, and emotional stress. Reintroduction helps ease these limitations while preserving health improvements.

4. **Empowering Self-Awareness:**
    - By carefully monitoring how foods affect the body, individuals gain a deeper understanding of their unique needs and can make informed choices about their diet moving forward.

The reintroduction phase is not merely about adding foods back—it's about striking a balance between healing and flexibility, creating a sustainable lifestyle that supports long-term health.

Systematic Reintroduction Process

The success of the reintroduction phase depends on a methodical approach. Rushing or reintroducing multiple foods simultaneously can obscure results and undo progress. The following step-by-step guide ensures a safe and effective process:

1. Preparation and Planning

Before beginning reintroduction, it's important to:

- **Assess Your Progress:** Ensure that symptoms have stabilized or improved significantly during the elimination phase. Lingering or severe symptoms may indicate the need for a longer elimination period.
- **Keep a Food Journal:** Maintain a detailed record of foods reintroduced, portion sizes, and any symptoms experienced. This will help identify patterns and reactions over time.
- **Prioritize Foods:** Decide which foods to reintroduce first based on their nutritional value, cultural importance, or personal preference.

2. Choose One Food at a Time

- Select a single food to reintroduce. Start with foods that are least likely to cause a reaction, such as ghee or egg yolks. Avoid starting with highly allergenic or inflammatory foods like gluten or dairy.
- Begin with a small portion (e.g., 1 teaspoon of ghee or a bite of egg yolk) and monitor for reactions over the next 15–30 minutes. If no symptoms occur, increase the portion gradually over the course of the da

3. Monitor for Symptoms

- Observe your body for any signs of adverse reactions over the next **72 hours**. Common symptoms to watch for include:
    - Digestive issues (bloating, gas, diarrhea, or constipation)
    - Skin reactions (rash, itching, or hives)
    - Joint pain or stiffness
    - Fatigue or brain fog
    - Respiratory issues (nasal congestion, wheezing)

If no symptoms arise, the food is likely safe to include in your diet. If symptoms occur, the food should be eliminated again, and reintroduction may be retried after additional healing.

4. Wait Before Reintroducing the Next Food

- Allow at least **5-7 days** between reintroducing foods to ensure that any delayed reactions are not missed. This waiting period also gives your body time to recover from potential symptoms before introducing a new food.

5. Reintroduce Foods in Categories

To streamline the process, foods can be reintroduced in groups based on their likelihood of causing reactions.

1. **Foods Least Likely to Trigger Symptoms:**
   - Ghee, egg yolks, fermented foods (e.g., sauerkraut), and certain seeds (e.g., chia, flax).
2. **Moderately Challenging Foods:**
   - Egg whites, nuts (e.g., almonds, walnuts), and nightshades (e.g., tomatoes, bell peppers).
3. **Highly Allergenic Foods:**
   - Dairy (milk, cheese), gluten-containing grains (wheat, barley, rye), and processed foods with additives.

Reintroducing foods in this order minimizes the risk of overwhelming the immune system and helps build confidence in the process.

6. Adjust Based on Individual Tolerance

- If a food triggers mild symptoms, consider reintroducing it again in smaller portions after several weeks of additional healing. Some foods may require multiple attempts before tolerance improves.
- Understand that not all foods will be tolerated, and that's okay. The reintroduction process is about learning what works for your unique body.

Tips for Success

1. **Stay Patient and Flexible:** Healing is not linear, and the reintroduction phase may take time. Listen to your body and adjust the pace as needed.
2. **Avoid Emotional Reactions:** If a food triggers symptoms, don't view it as a failure. Focus on the progress you've made and move forward with the process.
3. **Seek Professional Guidance:** Working with a nutritionist or healthcare provider experienced in AIP can provide additional

support and ensure that your diet remains balanced and nutrient-dense.

The reintroduction phase is a powerful opportunity to tailor the Autoimmune Protocol to your unique needs. By following a systematic and thoughtful process, you can expand your diet, reduce unnecessary restrictions, and create a sustainable approach to managing autoimmune conditions. The knowledge gained through reintroduction empowers you to make informed dietary choices, supporting long-term health and well-being.

Monitoring and Identifying Food Sensitivities

Successfully navigating the reintroduction phase of the Autoimmune Protocol (AIP) hinges on your ability to monitor and identify food sensitivities. This process requires attentiveness, patience, and the willingness to embrace a trial-and-error approach. Here's a detailed guide on how to effectively monitor your body's responses and recognize potential triggers:

1. The Role of Food Journaling

A food journal is an indispensable tool for tracking your dietary experiments during the reintroduction phase. It helps document how your body responds to specific foods and provides clarity amidst what might otherwise feel like a confusing or overwhelming process.

- **What to Record:**
    - The food reintroduced (e.g., almonds, egg whites).
    - Portion size and preparation method.
    - Time of consumption.
    - Any physical, mental, or emotional symptoms observed (e.g., bloating, fatigue, irritability).

- Duration of symptoms and their intensity (mild, moderate, severe).
- **Benefits:**
  - Patterns and correlations between foods and symptoms become easier to identify.
  - It creates a reference point for future dietary adjustments.

2. Recognizing Symptoms of Food Sensitivities

Food sensitivities can manifest in various ways, sometimes hours or even days after consumption. Being aware of potential symptoms helps you better identify problematic foods.

- **Digestive Symptoms:**
  - Bloating, gas, diarrhea, or constipation.
  - Stomach cramps or nausea.
- **Skin Reactions:**
  - Hives, rashes, redness, or itching.
  - Eczema flare-ups.
- **Joint and Muscle Issues:**
  - Pain, stiffness, or swelling in joints.
  - Muscle fatigue or weakness.
- **Cognitive and Emotional Symptoms:**
  - Brain fog, difficulty concentrating, or forgetfulness.
  - Mood swings, irritability, or anxiety.
- **Other Reactions:**
  - Nasal congestion, sinus issues, or wheezing.
  - Unusual fatigue, headaches, or sleep disturbances.

3. Observing Patterns and Delayed Reactions

Food sensitivities are not always immediate. Some reactions may take up to 72 hours to appear, making it essential to monitor your body for several days after introducing a new food.

- **Immediate Reactions:** Occur within minutes to a few hours, such as stomach upset or a rash.
- **Delayed Reactions:** Take longer to surface and may include joint pain or fatigue experienced a day or two later.

By maintaining a consistent food journal and avoiding the temptation to reintroduce multiple foods simultaneously, you can pinpoint even the most subtle delayed reactions.

4. Managing Cross-Reactivity

Some foods share similar proteins, which can lead to cross-reactivity. For example, individuals sensitive to latex may also react to bananas or avocados. Understanding this concept can help you make more informed choices if a reaction occurs.

5. Avoiding False Positives

External factors such as stress, poor sleep, or hormonal fluctuations can mimic or exacerbate symptoms, leading to confusion about whether a food is truly triggering a reaction. To minimize this:

- Ensure you are in a stable state of health when reintroducing a food.
- Repeat the test for any food that triggers a mild or ambiguous reaction to confirm the sensitivity.

Personalizing Your Diet Post-Reintroduction

The ultimate goal of the AIP reintroduction phase is to transition into a personalized, nutrient-dense diet that supports your health while accommodating your unique sensitivities and preferences. This step requires integrating the knowledge gained during reintroduction into your daily life.

1. Identifying Safe Foods

Post-reintroduction, you'll have a clearer understanding of which foods your body tolerates well. These foods become the foundation of your diet.

- Emphasize nutrient-dense options such as lean proteins, colorful vegetables, healthy fats, and tolerated fruits.
- Rotate foods regularly to promote dietary diversity and prevent new sensitivities.

2. Establishing Trigger Awareness

Not all problematic foods need to be permanently avoided. Some may cause mild reactions that are manageable in small quantities or when consumed infrequently.

- Create a list of "occasional foods" that you can tolerate in limited amounts without significant symptoms.
- Develop strategies to avoid or minimize accidental exposure to more severe triggers, such as reading ingredient labels carefully or planning ahead when dining out.

3. Striking a Balance Between Healing and Flexibility

Personalization doesn't mean perfection. A balanced diet is one that prioritizes healing while also allowing room for flexibility and enjoyment.

- **Social Occasions:** Learn how to navigate situations like holidays or dining out while maintaining your dietary boundaries. For example, bring your own dish to gatherings or research restaurants in advance.
- **Mindful Eating:** Practice being present during meals, savoring flavors, and listening to your body's hunger and satiety cues.

4. Reassessing Over Time

The personalization process is not static. Over time, as your body continues to heal, you may find that you tolerate foods that were once problematic. Periodically reassess foods that were initially excluded to determine if they can now be included.

5. Working with Professionals

For more complex cases, working with a functional medicine practitioner or registered dietitian can provide additional support. Professionals can guide you through reintroductions, address nutrient deficiencies, and create tailored meal plans to meet your health goals.

Monitoring and identifying food sensitivities during the reintroduction phase is a transformative process that equips you with the tools to create a personalized diet. By understanding your body's unique responses, you can build a lifestyle that balances health, flexibility, and enjoyment, empowering you to live vibrantly despite autoimmune challenges.

Meal Planning and Preparation

Implementing the Autoimmune Protocol (AIP) into your daily life begins with mastering meal planning and preparation. A well-organized approach to meals not only ensures that you stay on track but also makes the process enjoyable and sustainable. Here's how to seamlessly incorporate AIP principles into your kitchen and daily routine:

1. Building an AIP-Approved Pantry

Stocking your kitchen with AIP-compliant foods is the first step toward successful meal planning. Having the right ingredients on hand reduces temptation and simplifies cooking.

- **Staple Proteins**: Grass-fed beef, wild-caught fish, pasture-raised poultry, and organ meats.
- **Vegetables**: Leafy greens, cruciferous vegetables (e.g., broccoli, cauliflower), squashes, and root vegetables.
- **Fats**: Coconut oil, avocado oil, olive oil, and duck fat.
- **Snacks**: Dried fruits (unsweetened), coconut chips, or plantain chips (baked).
- **Seasonings**: Fresh herbs, garlic, ginger, and AIP-friendly spice blends (avoid nightshades like paprika or chili powder).

2. Weekly Meal Planning Tips

A structured meal plan minimizes stress and decision fatigue. Dedicate time each week to create a menu and grocery list that aligns with AIP guidelines.

- **Batch Cooking**: Prepare large portions of proteins, vegetables, and sides to store in the fridge or freezer for quick access. For example, roast a whole chicken and use it for salads, soups, or stir-fries throughout the week.
- **One-Pot Meals**: Soups, stews, and casseroles are AIP-friendly and save time on cooking and cleanup.
- **Balanced Plates**: Each meal should include a combination of protein, healthy fats, and a variety of vegetables for optimal nutrient intake.

3. Simplifying Preparation with Tools

Investing in kitchen tools can make cooking AIP meals more efficient.

- **Essentials:** A high-quality chef's knife, cutting board, and vegetable peeler.
- **Helpful Gadgets:** Slow cooker, pressure cooker, or food processor for faster meal prep.
- **Storage Solutions:** Glass containers for storing prepped ingredients or leftovers.

4. AIP Breakfast Ideas

Breakfast can be challenging on AIP due to the exclusion of eggs, grains, and dairy. Creative options include:

- Sweet potato hash with ground turkey and sautéed spinach.
- A smoothie made with coconut milk, avocado, and frozen berries.
- Leftovers from dinner (e.g., a small serving of roasted chicken and veggies).

5. Staying Inspired

To avoid meal monotony, experiment with new recipes and cuisines. Explore AIP cookbooks, blogs, or social media for fresh ideas that expand your culinary horizons.

Navigating Social Situations and Dining Out

Social gatherings and dining out can pose challenges for individuals following the Autoimmune Protocol. However, with some preparation and communication, you can maintain your dietary commitments while enjoying these experiences.

1. Preparing for Social Gatherings

Attending events where food is central doesn't have to derail your progress.

- **Communicate Ahead:** Let your host know about your dietary needs in advance. Offer to bring a dish that aligns with AIP so you'll have something to enjoy.
- **Eat Beforehand:** If you're unsure about the menu, eat a small, satisfying meal before the event to avoid hunger and temptation.
- **Focus on Connection:** Shift your attention away from food and toward meaningful interactions with friends and family.

2. Strategies for Dining Out

Dining at restaurants while adhering to AIP requires thoughtful planning and clear communication.

- **Research Ahead:** Look up menus online and identify AIP-friendly options before you go. Many restaurants offer grilled proteins and steamed vegetables that can be customized.
- **Ask Questions:** Don't hesitate to ask about ingredients, preparation methods, or possible substitutions. For instance, request olive oil instead of butter for cooking.
- **Customize Your Order:** Build a meal from side dishes if needed, such as pairing grilled chicken with a double serving of steamed broccoli or salad greens.

3. Managing Peer Pressure and Questions

Explaining your dietary choices can sometimes feel uncomfortable, but confidence and positivity go a long way.

- **Be Honest, but Brief:** A simple explanation like, "I'm following a specific protocol to improve my health," is often enough.

- **Stay Positive:** Frame your choices as something you're excited about, rather than something restrictive. For example, "I've been feeling so much better eating this way."
- **Redirect the Conversation:** Shift focus by asking others about their own health or interests.

4. Emergency Snacks and Meals

Having backup options can save the day in situations where AIP-compliant foods aren't available.

- **Travel Snacks:** Bring portable items like dried meat, coconut flakes, or sliced vegetables when attending events or traveling.
- **Frozen Meals:** Keep a stash of AIP-approved meals in your freezer for quick reheating on busy days.

Implementing AIP into your daily life is a manageable and rewarding process when approached with preparation and adaptability. By mastering meal planning, equipping your kitchen with essentials, and developing strategies for social situations, you can maintain your commitment to healing without feeling deprived. The key lies in being proactive, staying flexible, and prioritizing your well-being at every step.

Budget-Friendly AIP Strategies

Following the Autoimmune Protocol (AIP) doesn't have to break the bank. With careful planning, strategic shopping, and creative use of ingredients, you can adhere to this nutrient-rich dietary approach while staying within your financial means. Here's how to implement AIP on a budget without compromising on quality or health:

1. Prioritize Whole, Unprocessed Foods

The foundation of AIP is built on fresh, whole foods, which can be cost-effective if you shop smartly.

- **Focus on Basics:** Buy affordable staples like sweet potatoes, carrots, cabbage, ground meats, and canned fish (e.g., sardines or salmon).
- **Seasonal Produce:** Choose fruits and vegetables that are in season for better prices and peak flavor. Visit local farmers' markets or join community-supported agriculture (CSA) programs.
- **Frozen Options:** Frozen vegetables and fruits are often cheaper than fresh and just as nutritious.

2. Buy in Bulk

Purchasing certain items in bulk can lead to significant savings.

- **Pantry Staples:** Look for deals on coconut flour, cassava flour, or coconut milk.
- **Proteins:** Buy large quantities of meat or fish when on sale, then portion and freeze them for later use.
- **Storage:** Invest in freezer-safe bags or containers to keep bulk items fresh.

3. Plan and Prep Meals

Meal planning reduces food waste and ensures you stick to your budget.

- **Batch Cooking:** Prepare large quantities of soups, stews, or roasted vegetables, which can be reheated throughout the week.
- **Leftovers:** Repurpose leftovers into new meals to minimize waste (e.g., roast chicken one night, then use the leftover meat for soup or salad).
- **One-Pot Meals:** Economical and easy to prepare, these meals save time and reduce cleanup.

4. DIY Convenience Foods

Pre-packaged AIP-friendly snacks and condiments can be expensive. Making your own at home is both cost-effective and healthier.

- **Bone Broth:** Save chicken or beef bones to make nutrient-dense broth.
- **Snack Bars:** Create homemade bars using dates, coconut, and compliant seeds.
- **AIP Condiments:** Prepare your own salad dressings, marinades, and sauces using fresh ingredients.

5. Embrace Affordable Protein Sources

Protein is a cornerstone of the AIP diet but can be costly. Opt for budget-friendly options.

- **Organ Meats:** Liver and heart are nutrient-dense, AIP-compliant, and much cheaper than muscle meats.
- **Egg-Free Alternatives:** Canned fish like tuna or sardines offer a great source of omega-3s.
- **Plant-Based Options:** Incorporate moderate amounts of AIP-friendly plant proteins like coconut or tiger nuts.

6. Avoid Expensive AIP "Extras"

While specialty AIP products can be tempting, they aren't necessary. Focus on the basics and reserve extra spending for occasional treats.

- **Skip Pre-Made Mixes:** Opt for simple homemade recipes instead of buying pre-made AIP pancake or bread mixes.
- **Limit Superfoods:** While items like collagen powder are beneficial, they are not essential to the protocol.

Maintaining Motivation and Consistency

Consistency is the key to achieving the long-term health benefits of the Autoimmune Protocol. While sticking to such a comprehensive dietary and lifestyle regimen can be challenging, cultivating the right mindset and habits can help you stay motivated and committed.

1. Set Clear Goals

Begin by identifying your primary reasons for adopting AIP. These goals will serve as powerful motivators during moments of doubt.

- **Health Goals:** Examples include reducing inflammation, alleviating symptoms, or improving energy levels.
- **Personal Goals:** Beyond health, you may aim to learn more about your body's unique sensitivities or foster a sustainable way of eating.

2. Celebrate Small Wins

Acknowledge and celebrate milestones to keep yourself motivated.

- **Health Improvements:** Recognize progress, such as better sleep, fewer flare-ups, or increased energy.
- **Dietary Successes:** Appreciate your ability to stick to AIP in challenging situations, like dining out or attending social events.

3. Build a Support System

Surrounding yourself with supportive individuals can make a significant difference.

- **Family and Friends:** Share your journey with loved ones to help them understand and respect your choices.

- **Online Communities:** Join AIP forums or social media groups to connect with others, exchange recipes, and share experiences.

4. Embrace Variety and Creativity

A repetitive diet can lead to boredom and reduced adherence.

- **Experiment with Recipes:** Try new AIP-friendly recipes or explore different cuisines that align with the protocol.
- **Rotate Foods:** Avoid eating the same items daily to reduce the risk of developing new sensitivities and to keep meals exciting.

5. Practice Mindfulness

Mindfulness helps you stay present and engaged with your dietary and lifestyle choices.

- **Mindful Eating:** Focus on the sensory experience of eating—taste, texture, and aroma.
- **Stress Reduction:** Incorporate practices like yoga, meditation, or deep breathing to support emotional well-being.

6. Plan for Challenges

Anticipate obstacles and develop strategies to overcome them.

- **Travel and Dining Out:** Pack compliant snacks, research AIP-friendly restaurants, or bring your own meals.
- **Cravings:** Combat cravings with satisfying AIP-compliant alternatives or by addressing the emotional triggers behind them.

7. Reassess and Adjust

As your body heals, you may need to revisit and modify your approach.

- **Evaluate Progress**: Periodically reflect on how your symptoms and overall well-being have improved.
- **Tweak as Needed**: Adjust your diet or lifestyle practices based on new insights or changing needs.

Stress Management Techniques

Stress plays a critical role in the development and progression of autoimmune diseases. When left unchecked, chronic stress can exacerbate inflammation, disrupt immune function, and hinder your body's ability to heal. Incorporating effective stress management techniques alongside the

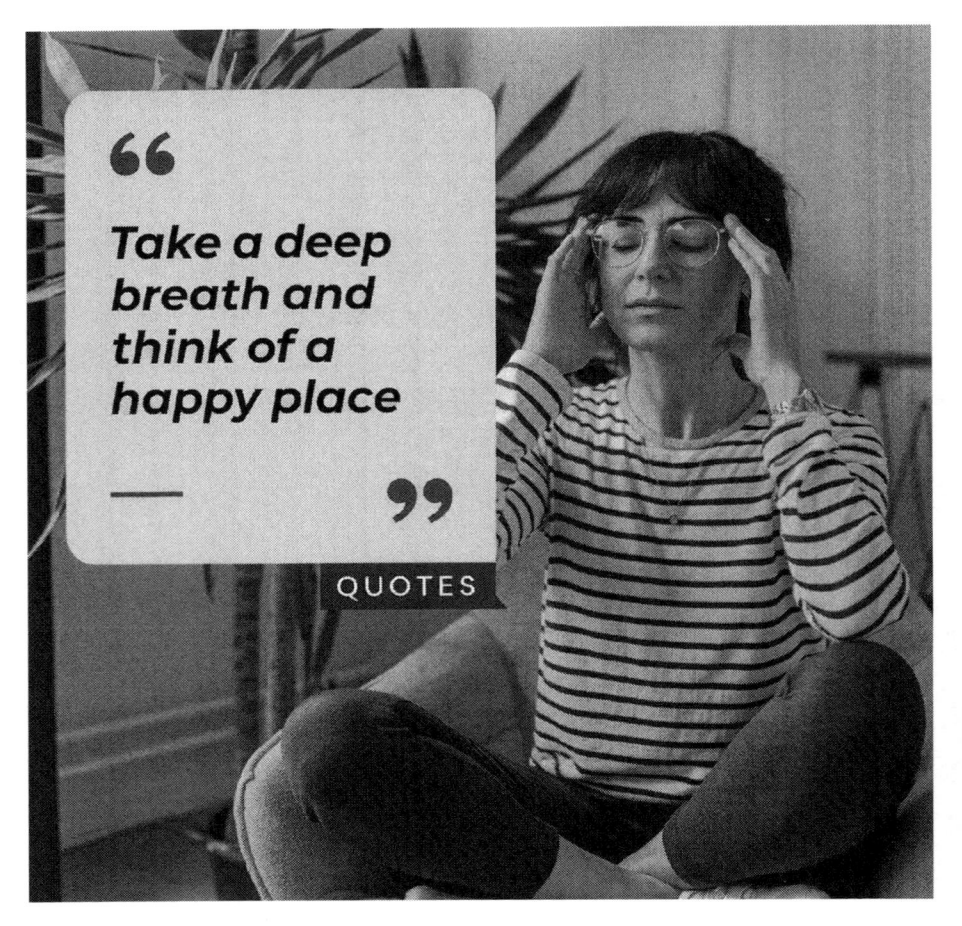

Autoimmune Protocol (AIP) can help create a balanced and healing environment for your body.

1. Understand the Stress-Immune Connection

To effectively manage stress, it's important to understand its impact on your health:

- **Chronic Stress:** Activates the hypothalamic-pituitary-adrenal (HPA) axis, leading to elevated cortisol levels that weaken the immune system over time.
- **Inflammation:** Prolonged stress can promote inflammation, a driving factor in autoimmune conditions.
- **Gut-Brain Axis:** Stress disrupts gut health, impairing digestion and affecting the microbiome, which is central to AIP's principles.

2. Techniques to Manage Stress

- **Mindfulness Meditation:**
    - Practicing mindfulness helps you stay present and reduces anxiety. Even a few minutes a day can lower stress hormones and improve mental clarity.
    - Start with deep breathing exercises or guided meditations. Apps like Calm or Headspace offer beginner-friendly options.
- **Yoga and Stretching:**
    - Yoga combines movement, breathwork, and meditation, reducing stress while promoting physical flexibility and strength.

- o Gentle, restorative yoga is particularly beneficial for individuals with autoimmune conditions.
- **Journaling:**
  - o Writing about your thoughts and feelings can help process emotions and release mental tension.
  - o Consider maintaining a gratitude journal to focus on positive aspects of your life.
- **Nature Therapy:**
  - o Spending time outdoors, whether through walking, hiking, or gardening, can significantly lower cortisol levels and promote a sense of calm.
- **Social Support:**
  - o Building a network of supportive friends, family, or AIP communities provides emotional relief and practical encouragement during challenging times.

3. Tailoring Stress Management to Your Needs

- Experiment with different techniques to find what resonates with you.
- Schedule stress-relief activities into your daily routine, just as you would a meal or a meeting.
- Listen to your body and recognize when stress is manifesting physically or emotionally, then take proactive steps to address it.

The Importance of Quality Sleep

Sleep is a cornerstone of health, especially for those managing autoimmune diseases. Restorative sleep allows the body to repair, regulate inflammation, and optimize immune function, all of which are crucial for the success of the AIP lifestyle.

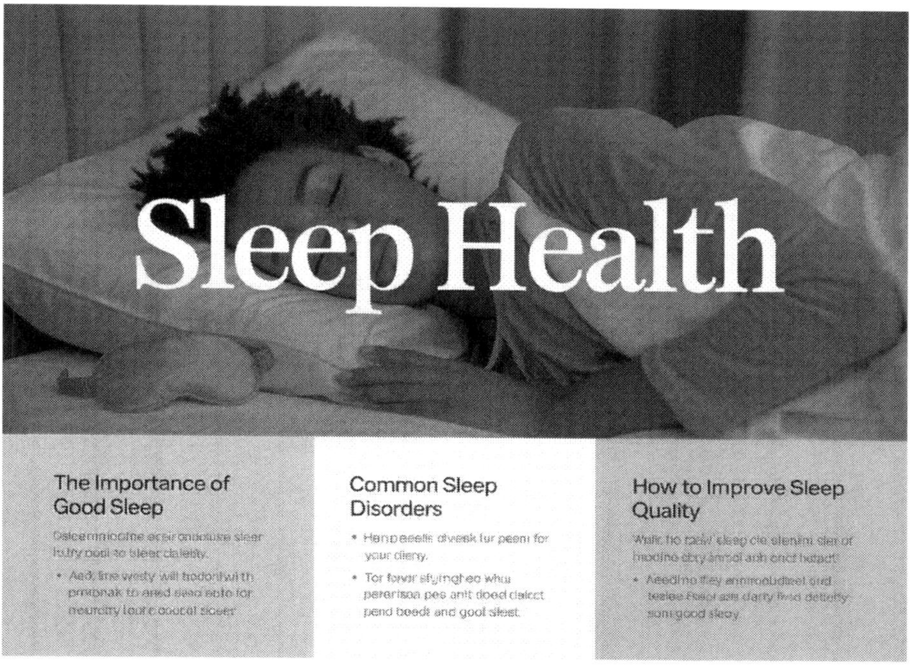
Sleep Health
The Importance of Good Sleep
Common Sleep Disorders
How to Improve Sleep Quality

1. The Science of Sleep and Autoimmunity

- **Inflammation Control**: During deep sleep, the body regulates inflammatory responses, reducing the severity of autoimmune symptoms.
- **Immune Function**: Sleep enhances the production of T-cells and cytokines, which are essential for immune system balance.
- **Hormonal Regulation**: Proper sleep maintains a healthy balance of hormones like cortisol and melatonin, which influence immune health and stress levels.

2. Strategies for Improving Sleep Quality

- **Establish a Sleep Routine:**

- Go to bed and wake up at the same time every day, even on weekends.
- Create a calming pre-sleep ritual, such as reading, stretching, or meditating.
- **Optimize Your Sleep Environment:**
  - Keep your bedroom dark, quiet, and cool. Use blackout curtains or a white noise machine if needed.
  - Invest in a comfortable mattress and pillows that support restful sleep.
- **Limit Screen Time:**
  - Blue light from phones, tablets, and computers disrupts melatonin production, making it harder to fall asleep.
  - Avoid screens at least 1–2 hours before bedtime or use blue light-blocking glasses.
- **Focus on Nutrition:**
  - Incorporate AIP-friendly foods that promote sleep, such as fatty fish, leafy greens, and magnesium-rich vegetables.
  - Avoid stimulants like caffeine or sugar, especially in the afternoon and evening.
- **Exercise Regularly:**
  - Physical activity during the day promotes better sleep at night. Choose gentle exercises like walking, swimming, or yoga to avoid overexertion.
- **Manage Stress Before Bed:**
  - Practice relaxation techniques, such as deep breathing or progressive muscle relaxation, to calm your mind and body.

3. Recognizing and Addressing Sleep Disorders

If you struggle with persistent sleep issues, it's essential to identify potential underlying causes:

- **Insomnia:** Difficulty falling or staying asleep may stem from stress, poor sleep hygiene, or medical conditions.
- **Sleep Apnea:** This disorder disrupts breathing during sleep and can worsen autoimmune symptoms. Consult a healthcare provider if you suspect this issue.
- **Chronic Pain:** If autoimmune-related pain disrupts your sleep, discuss pain management strategies with your doctor.

Integrating Stress and Sleep into AIP

Combining effective stress management and quality sleep practices with the Autoimmune Protocol creates a powerful synergy for healing. By reducing stress and optimizing sleep, you enhance your body's ability to restore balance, minimize inflammation, and promote long-term wellness. Remember, these lifestyle factors are just as vital as dietary changes in your journey to overcoming autoimmunity.

Incorporating Appropriate Physical Activity

Physical activity is a vital component of overall health, but for individuals managing autoimmune conditions, it requires careful consideration. The right type and intensity of exercise can reduce inflammation, improve circulation, and enhance mood. However, overexertion can exacerbate symptoms and lead to flare-ups. Incorporating appropriate physical activity alongside the Autoimmune Protocol (AIP) supports a balanced approach to healing and recovery.

1. Understanding the Role of Exercise in Autoimmunity

- **Inflammation Reduction:** Moderate exercise helps regulate inflammatory markers, reducing chronic inflammation associated with autoimmune conditions.

- **Immune System Modulation:** Regular physical activity strengthens the immune system, promoting a balanced response rather than an overactive, self-targeting one.
- **Improved Mental Health:** Exercise reduces stress and anxiety, which can worsen autoimmune symptoms.

2. Choosing the Right Type of Exercise

Autoimmune conditions often require a tailored approach to physical activity, focusing on gentle, restorative movements rather than high-intensity workouts.

- **Low-Impact Activities:**
  - Walking: A simple, accessible way to boost circulation and mood.
  - Swimming: Reduces joint strain while offering a full-body workout.
  - Cycling: Provides cardiovascular benefits with minimal impact on joints.
- **Mind-Body Exercises:**
  - Yoga: Improves flexibility, balance, and relaxation, while calming the nervous system.
  - Tai Chi: Combines slow, deliberate movements with deep breathing, promoting stress relief and joint mobility.
  - Pilates: Builds core strength and improves posture, which can alleviate pain and tension.
- **Strength Training:**
  - Light resistance exercises can help maintain muscle mass and bone density, especially for those with joint or mobility issues.
- **Stretching and Mobility Work:**
  - Daily stretching keeps muscles flexible and reduces stiffness, a common issue in autoimmune conditions.

3. Finding the Right Balance

- **Start Slow:** Begin with short, low-intensity sessions and gradually increase duration and intensity as your body adapts.
- **Listen to Your Body:** Rest on days when fatigue or pain is high. Pushing through discomfort can worsen symptoms.
- **Focus on Consistency:** Regular, gentle exercise is more beneficial than sporadic, intense workouts. Aim for 20–30 minutes of movement most days of the week.

4. Monitoring Progress and Adjusting

- Track your energy levels and symptom changes to identify which activities work best for you.
- Consult a physical therapist or personal trainer with experience in autoimmune conditions for personalized guidance.
- Remember that exercise is not a one-size-fits-all solution—what works for someone else may not be ideal for you.

Building a Supportive Community

Managing an autoimmune condition can often feel isolating. Building a supportive community offers emotional encouragement, practical advice, and a sense of belonging, all of which are essential for long-term success with the Autoimmune Protocol.

1. The Importance of Support Systems

- **Emotional Well-being:** Sharing experiences and challenges with others reduces feelings of loneliness and anxiety.
- **Motivation:** A supportive community can help you stay committed to AIP, especially during difficult periods.
- **Learning Opportunities:** Interacting with others on similar journeys provides access to tips, recipes, and success stories.

2. Creating Your Support Network

Building a strong community starts with identifying people and resources that align with your goals and values:

- **Family and Friends:**
    - Educate your loved ones about AIP so they can better understand your dietary and lifestyle choices.
    - Involve them in meal planning or invite them to join you in gentle physical activities.
- **Online Communities:**
    - Join AIP-specific groups on social media platforms or forums where you can connect with others navigating similar challenges.
    - Share your progress, ask questions, and seek advice from a diverse group of individuals.
- **Local Support Groups:**
    - Look for autoimmune-focused support groups or workshops in your area.
    - Participating in face-to-face interactions fosters deeper connections.
- **Healthcare Team:**
    - Work closely with healthcare providers who understand your condition and support AIP principles.
    - A nutritionist or dietitian can offer guidance and accountability.
- **Accountability Partners:**
    - Find a friend, family member, or fellow AIP participant to help you stay on track and celebrate milestones.

3. Maintaining and Nurturing Your Community

- **Engage Regularly**: Actively participate in discussions, whether online or in person, to build lasting relationships.
- **Offer Support**: Share your knowledge and encouragement with others. Helping someone else can reinforce your own commitment to AIP.
- **Respect Individual Journeys**: Remember that everyone's autoimmune journey is unique. Avoid comparisons and focus on your progress.

Integrating Exercise and Community into AIP

Combining appropriate physical activity with a supportive community creates a holistic approach to managing autoimmune conditions. Movement nurtures the body, while a network of supportive individuals uplifts the mind and spirit. Together, these elements amplify the benefits of the Autoimmune Protocol, fostering resilience, connection, and healing.

Medical Research and Evidence Supporting AIP

The Autoimmune Protocol (AIP) is rooted in scientific principles and bolstered by emerging research that highlights its effectiveness in managing autoimmune conditions. This chapter explores the body of evidence supporting AIP, focusing on clinical studies and their findings regarding specific autoimmune diseases.

Overview of Clinical Studies

Recent research has shed light on the impact of dietary and lifestyle changes on autoimmune disease management. While large-scale studies are still limited, the existing data consistently indicate that AIP has significant potential to reduce inflammation, alleviate symptoms, and improve quality of life for individuals with autoimmune disorders.

Key findings include:

- **Symptom Reduction:** Studies show that individuals following AIP report improvements in pain, fatigue, and digestive issues.
- **Inflammatory Markers:** AIP has been linked to reductions in markers like C-reactive protein (CRP), indicating lower inflammation.
- **Gut Health Improvements:** Many studies highlight AIP's role in restoring gut integrity and supporting a healthy microbiome, essential for autoimmune health.

Inflammatory Bowel Disease (IBD)

Inflammatory Bowel Disease, which includes Crohn's disease and ulcerative colitis, is characterized by chronic inflammation of the gastrointestinal tract. Research has demonstrated that AIP can be an effective tool for managing these conditions.

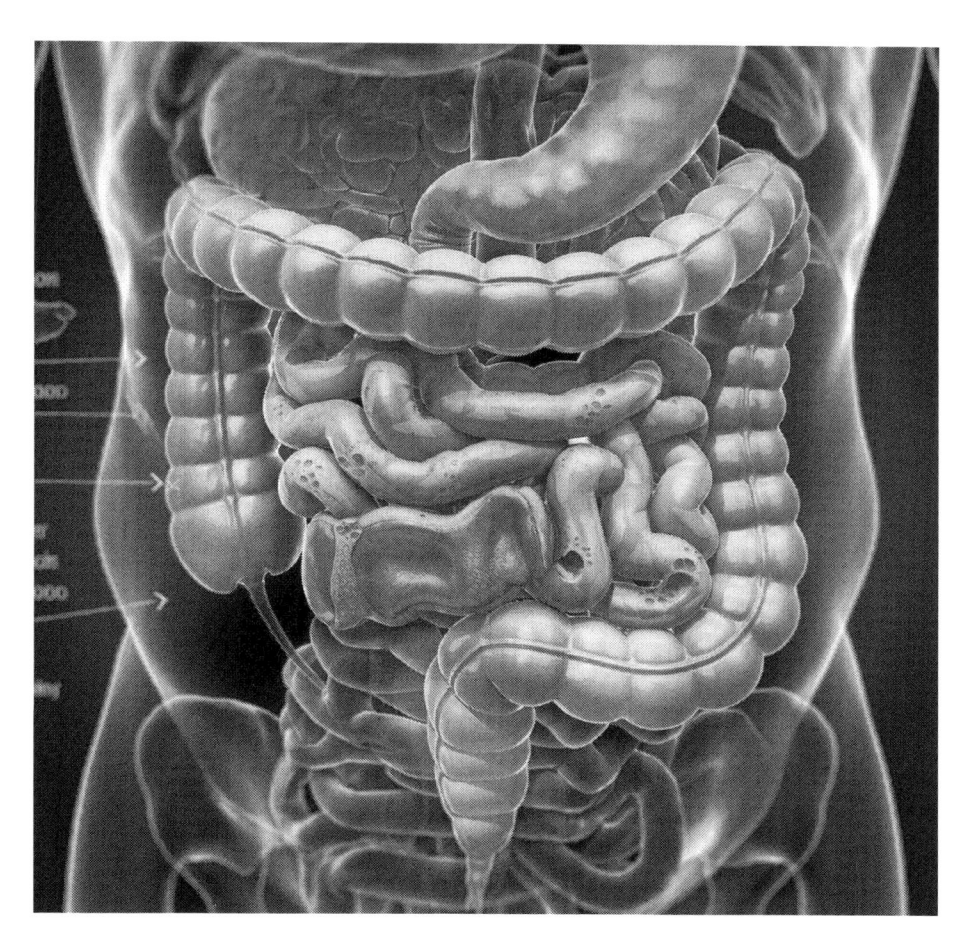

- **Clinical Evidence:**
    - A 2017 study published in the journal *Inflammatory Bowel Diseases* evaluated AIP in patients with Crohn's disease and ulcerative colitis.

- o Over 6 weeks, participants followed the AIP elimination phase, leading to an 80% clinical remission rate.
- o Improvements were observed in gut symptoms, inflammatory markers, and overall quality of life.
- **Mechanisms of Action:**
  - o AIP helps repair the intestinal lining, addressing "leaky gut," a common issue in IBD.
  - o The protocol reduces inflammatory triggers, such as gluten, processed foods, and dairy, which are known to aggravate gut inflammation.

Hashimoto's Thyroiditis

Hashimoto's Thyroiditis, the leading cause of hypothyroidism, involves an autoimmune attack on the thyroid gland. AIP has been found to support thyroid health by addressing underlying inflammation and immune dysregulation.

- **Clinical Evidence:**
  - o Studies have highlighted improvements in thyroid hormone levels and symptom reduction in individuals with Hashimoto's who adhere to AIP.
  - o Patient-reported outcomes indicate reduced fatigue, brain fog, and joint pain.
- **Key Benefits of AIP for Hashimoto's:**
  - o Supports nutrient-dense foods rich in iodine, selenium, and zinc, which are crucial for thyroid health.
  - o Eliminates inflammatory foods that can exacerbate autoimmune activity against the thyroid.
  - o Enhances gut health, addressing the gut-thyroid connection.

Rheumatoid Arthritis (RA)

Rheumatoid Arthritis is an autoimmune condition characterized by chronic joint inflammation and pain. Research suggests that AIP can play a significant role in reducing RA symptoms and improving joint health.

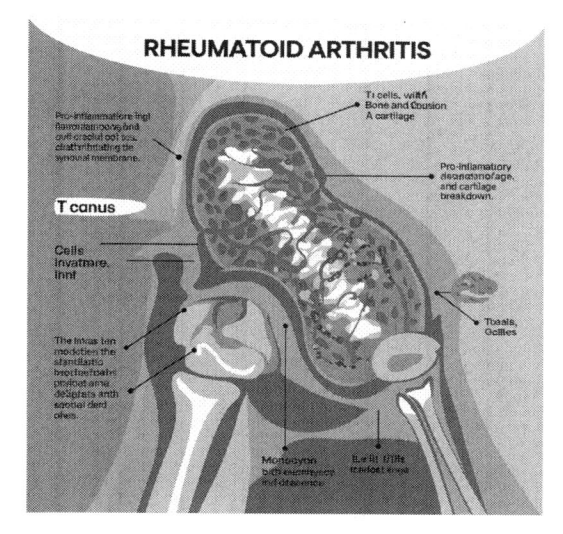

- **Clinical Evidence:**
    - A small but compelling body of evidence shows that individuals with RA experience reductions in joint pain, stiffness, and swelling after adopting AIP.
    - Improvements in inflammatory markers like CRP and ESR (erythrocyte sedimentation rate) have also been observed.
- **Mechanisms of Action:**
    - AIP removes common dietary triggers, such as refined sugars and nightshades, which can worsen joint inflammation.
    - It incorporates anti-inflammatory foods like omega-3-rich fish, leafy greens, and bone broth, which promote joint repair and reduce inflammation.

Broader Implications of AIP in Autoimmune Disease

Beyond these specific conditions, AIP has shown promise in managing a wide range of autoimmune diseases, including multiple sclerosis, lupus, and psoriasis. While more research is needed, the growing body of evidence underscores the protocol's potential to:

- Address systemic inflammation.
- Restore immune balance.
- Enhance overall well-being through a nutrient-dense diet and lifestyle adjustments.

Challenges in Medical Research and the Path Forward

While the existing research is promising, challenges remain:

- **Limited Large-Scale Studies:** Most studies on AIP involve small sample sizes, highlighting the need for broader clinical trials.
- **Long-Term Data:** Longitudinal studies are required to assess the sustained benefits of AIP over time.
- **Interdisciplinary Collaboration:** Greater integration of dietary and lifestyle interventions into conventional medical research can expand the understanding of AIP's potential.

The Autoimmune Protocol is gaining recognition as a powerful tool for managing autoimmune diseases. Backed by growing clinical evidence, AIP offers hope to individuals seeking natural, science-based approaches to healing. By addressing the root causes of autoimmunity—chronic inflammation, gut health, and immune dysregulation—AIP empowers individuals to take charge of their health and improve their quality of life.

Interpreting Research Findings

Interpreting the results of studies on the Autoimmune Protocol (AIP) requires careful consideration of various factors, including the scope of the study, the methodologies used, and the context in which the findings are presented. While the available research indicates positive outcomes for individuals with autoimmune diseases, the interpretation of these findings is still evolving, and further research is necessary to draw more definitive conclusions.

1. Understanding the Study Design and Scope

- **Study Size and Population:** Many studies investigating AIP are limited in size and scope, often focusing on small sample groups. This can impact the generalizability of the results. Larger, multi-center studies are needed to confirm the findings and provide a broader understanding of the protocol's efficacy.
- **Control Groups and Randomization:** AIP studies often lack control groups or randomization, which are essential components of robust clinical trials. Without these controls, it is difficult to isolate the effect of the AIP from other factors that could influence results, such as concurrent treatments or lifestyle changes.
- **Duration of Studies:** The majority of AIP-related studies are short-term, ranging from a few weeks to a few months. Longer-term studies are essential to assess the sustainability of the benefits observed and to determine whether AIP can provide lasting improvements in autoimmune conditions.

2. Analyzing Results: Benefits and Limitations

While current studies suggest that AIP can provide symptom relief and reduce inflammation in individuals with autoimmune diseases, there are inherent limitations that must be considered in interpreting the findings:

- **Symptom Management vs. Disease Remission:** Many studies show that AIP helps individuals manage symptoms such as fatigue, joint pain, and digestive issues. However, it's crucial to differentiate between symptom relief and disease remission. Long-term disease outcomes, including flare-ups and progression of the disease, are less well-documented.
- **Variation in Outcomes:** Individual responses to AIP can vary significantly. Factors such as the specific autoimmune disease, the severity of the condition, the individual's adherence to the protocol,

and genetic predispositions all play a role in the overall effectiveness of the diet. As such, not all participants may experience the same level of improvement.

- **Holistic Approach:** AIP emphasizes not just dietary changes but also lifestyle modifications such as stress management and sleep optimization. Research findings often do not isolate the effects of AIP diet alone, making it difficult to assess how much of the improvement is directly attributed to diet versus lifestyle changes.

3. The Importance of Patient-Reported Outcomes

In many studies on AIP, patient-reported outcomes (PROs) are central to understanding the protocol's impact. These self-reported measures, such as improvements in quality of life, fatigue levels, and pain, provide valuable insight into the everyday benefits of AIP. However, it is important to remember that PROs are subjective and may not always align with clinical biomarkers or other objective measures of health.

Future Directions in AIP Research

The potential for AIP to revolutionize the management of autoimmune diseases is exciting, but future research must address existing gaps and refine our understanding of its effectiveness. Several areas of focus will be critical in advancing AIP research and providing clearer evidence to guide its clinical use.

1. Large-Scale Clinical Trials

- **Randomized Controlled Trials (RCTs):** The gold standard in clinical research, RCTs can provide high-quality data on the efficacy of AIP in treating autoimmune diseases. By comparing AIP to standard treatments or placebos, researchers can better isolate the effects of the protocol and confirm its benefits.

- **Multicenter Studies:** Collaborations between research institutions across different geographical locations will help expand the diversity of participants and make findings more applicable to various populations.
- **Long-Term Follow-Up:** To understand whether the benefits of AIP are sustainable over time, long-term follow-up studies are essential. This will also allow researchers to assess whether the diet has long-lasting effects on disease progression.

2. Mechanisms of Action

Understanding the underlying mechanisms that make AIP effective is crucial for validating its use in autoimmune disease management. Future research should focus on:

- **Gut-Immune System Interactions:** Given AIP's emphasis on gut health, more studies are needed to explore how specific foods or food groups influence the gut microbiome and immune function. Researchers should focus on understanding how eliminating certain foods affects the gut's ability to modulate immune responses.
- **Inflammatory Pathways:** Further research is required to determine how AIP modulates specific inflammatory pathways involved in autoimmune diseases. Investigating inflammatory markers and cytokines before and after AIP intervention will provide greater clarity on how the protocol affects inflammation at the molecular level.
- **Nutrient Absorption:** Exploring how the AIP diet influences the absorption of key nutrients—such as vitamin D, omega-3 fatty acids, and selenium—will contribute to a better understanding of its impact on immune health.

3. Personalized Approaches to AIP

Given that autoimmune conditions are diverse and multifactorial, future research should explore personalized versions of AIP tailored to the needs of individual patients. Research could focus on:

- **Genetic Factors:** Understanding how genetic predispositions to autoimmune diseases interact with AIP could help identify which individuals are most likely to benefit from the protocol.
- **Food Sensitivity Testing:** Investigating the use of food sensitivity testing and its integration into AIP will help identify which foods should be avoided on an individual basis, allowing for a more tailored approach to diet.
- **Combination Therapies:** Research could also examine the synergy between AIP and other therapies, including conventional medications, to determine the most effective treatment plans for autoimmune diseases.

4. Integration of AIP into Conventional Medical Practice

For AIP to become widely accepted as a treatment option for autoimmune diseases, further research is needed to integrate it into the mainstream medical framework. This includes:

- **Collaboration Between Dietitians, Physicians, and Researchers:** Collaborative efforts between healthcare professionals will ensure that AIP is used in a manner that complements existing treatments and is personalized to the needs of the patient.
- **Creating Guidelines and Protocols:** As evidence supporting AIP grows, clinical guidelines should be developed to help healthcare providers incorporate AIP into patient care plans. These guidelines would provide best practices for physicians and dietitians in supporting patients through the AIP process.

While the Autoimmune Protocol has shown promise in managing autoimmune diseases, more rigorous and extensive research is needed to fully understand its potential and limitations. The future of AIP research will focus on large-scale clinical trials, understanding the mechanisms behind its effects, personalized approaches, and integrating the protocol into conventional medical practice. As research continues to unfold, AIP could become a cornerstone in the management of autoimmune diseases, offering a natural and effective approach to healing.

Recipes and Meal Plans

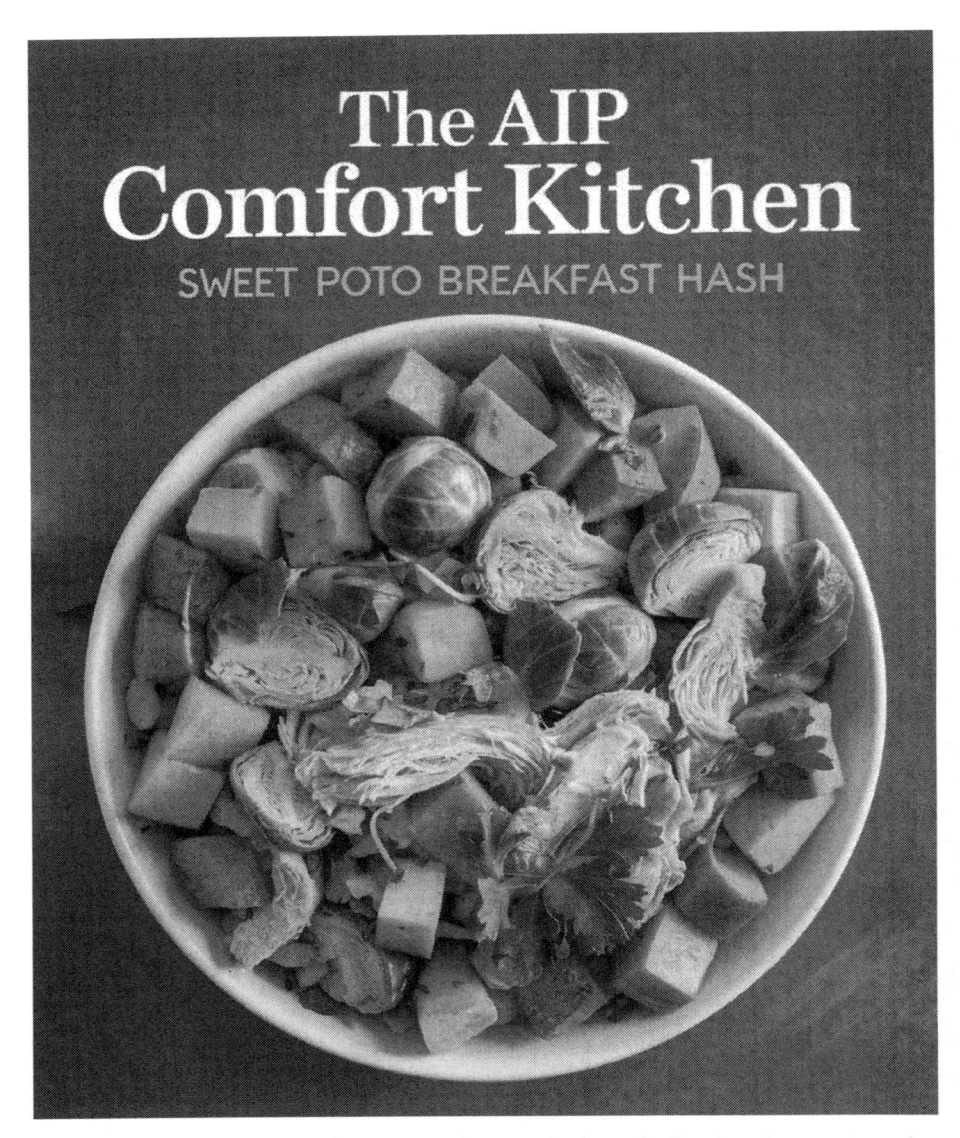

The AIP Comfort Kitchen
SWEET POTO BREAKFAST HASH

This chapter will provide you with practical tools for implementing the Autoimmune Protocol (AIP) into your everyday life. The recipes and meal plans featured here have been carefully curated to support healing, reduce inflammation, and nourish your body with nutrient-dense foods. Whether you're looking for a quick breakfast to start your day or a hearty dinner to unwind in the evening, these recipes will help you stay on track while still enjoying delicious, satisfying meals.

Breakfast Options

Starting your day with a nutritious breakfast is essential when following the AIP, as it helps to stabilize blood sugar levels, provide energy, and set a positive tone for the rest of your meals. The following breakfast ideas are designed to be both satisfying and easy to prepare. They are rich in healthy fats, fiber, and protein, which support gut health and keep inflammation at bay.

1. AIP Porridge with Coconut and Cinnamon

This creamy porridge is perfect for a warm, comforting breakfast. It's made with coconut milk and nutrient-dense ingredients that help fuel your body with anti-inflammatory properties.

Ingredients:

- 1 cup coconut milk (full-fat, unsweetened)
- ½ cup unsweetened shredded coconut
- 2 tbsp ground flaxseeds
- 1 tsp cinnamon
- 1 tsp vanilla extract
- 1 tbsp chia seeds (optional)
- Fresh berries for topping

Instructions:

1. In a medium saucepan, combine coconut milk, shredded coconut, and cinnamon. Bring to a simmer over medium heat.

2. Add ground flaxseeds and chia seeds, stirring frequently until the mixture thickens (about 5 minutes).
3. Remove from heat and stir in vanilla extract.
4. Top with fresh berries and enjoy!

2. Sweet Potato Hash with Ground Turkey

Sweet potatoes are rich in beta-carotene and fiber, making them an excellent choice for breakfast when following AIP. Paired with ground turkey, this dish provides lean protein to keep you full longer.

Ingredients:

- 1 large sweet potato, peeled and diced
- 1 lb ground turkey
- 1 tbsp olive oil
- 1 tsp turmeric
- 1 tsp garlic powder
- Salt and pepper to taste
- Fresh parsley, chopped (for garnish)

Instructions:

1. Heat olive oil in a skillet over medium heat. Add the diced sweet potato and cook until softened (about 10 minutes), stirring occasionally.
2. In another pan, cook the ground turkey over medium heat, breaking it up with a spoon until browned.
3. Once the sweet potatoes are tender, add the turkey to the skillet with the sweet potatoes. Season with turmeric, garlic powder, salt, and pepper. Stir well.
4. Cook together for an additional 3–5 minutes.
5. Garnish with fresh parsley and serve hot.

3. Avocado and Smoked Salmon Salad

This AIP-friendly breakfast is rich in omega-3 fatty acids, which are known to combat inflammation and promote heart health. The healthy fats in avocado provide long-lasting energy and help absorb fat-soluble vitamins.

Ingredients:

- 1 ripe avocado, sliced
- 3 oz smoked salmon (make sure it's AIP-compliant)
- 1 handful of mixed greens (e.g., arugula, spinach, kale)
- 1 tbsp olive oil
- 1 tsp lemon juice
- Salt and pepper to taste

Instructions:

1. On a plate, arrange the sliced avocado and smoked salmon.
2. Toss mixed greens with olive oil and lemon juice, then place them on top of the avocado and salmon.
3. Season with salt and pepper to taste.
4. Enjoy immediately as a light yet fulfilling breakfast.

Lunch and Dinner Ideas

Lunch and dinner should be designed to keep you satisfied, balanced, and nourished throughout the day. These meal ideas emphasize whole, unprocessed ingredients that are easy to prepare and can be enjoyed in a variety of ways. Each meal is rich in fiber, healthy fats, and lean protein to promote gut health, reduce inflammation, and support recovery.

1. AIP Chicken and Vegetable Stir-Fry

This vibrant stir-fry is packed with fresh, colorful vegetables and lean chicken, providing a hearty, anti-inflammatory meal that's perfect for lunch or dinner.

Ingredients:

- 2 boneless, skinless chicken breasts, cut into bite-sized pieces
- 1 red bell pepper, thinly sliced
- 1 zucchini, sliced
- 1 cup broccoli florets
- 2 tbsp coconut oil
- 2 tbsp coconut aminos
- 1 tsp garlic powder
- 1 tsp ginger powder
- 1 tbsp sesame seeds (optional)

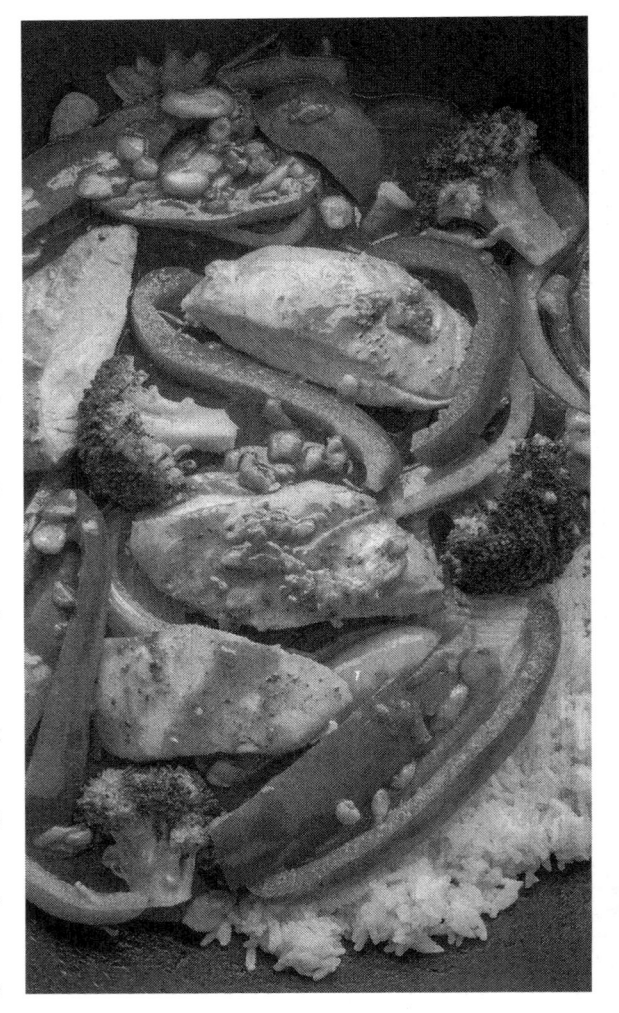

Instructions:

1. Heat coconut oil in a large skillet or wok over medium-high heat.
2. Add chicken pieces to the skillet and cook until browned and cooked through, about 7-8 minutes.

3. Add the bell pepper, zucchini, and broccoli to the skillet. Stir-fry for 4–5 minutes until the vegetables are tender but still crisp.
4. Pour in coconut aminos and season with garlic powder and ginger powder. Stir well.
5. Garnish with sesame seeds and serve immediately.

2. AIP Meatballs with Zucchini Noodles

AIP meatballs made with ground beef or turkey are a great source of protein, and when paired with zucchini noodles, they offer a delicious, low-carb meal that's both satisfying and nutrient-dense.

Ingredients:

- 1 lb ground beef or turkey
- 1 egg (optional)
- 1 tsp garlic powder
- 1 tsp onion powder
- 1 tsp dried oregano
- 1 zucchini, spiralized into noodles
- 1 tbsp olive oil
- 1 cup homemade or store-bought AIP-compliant marinara sauce (without nightshades)

Instructions:

1. Preheat your oven to 375°F (190°C).
2. In a bowl, combine ground meat, egg (optional), garlic powder, onion powder, and oregano. Roll into small meatballs and place them on a baking sheet.
3. Bake meatballs for 20 minutes or until cooked through.
4. While the meatballs are baking, heat olive oil in a large skillet over medium heat and sauté zucchini noodles for 3-4 minutes until tender.

5. Once the meatballs are ready, pour AIP-compliant marinara sauce over them and heat through.
6. Serve the meatballs over the zucchini noodles and enjoy!

3. Baked Salmon with Roasted Root Vegetables

Rich in omega-3 fatty acids and packed with antioxidants, this dish combines tender baked salmon with nutrient-rich root vegetables. It's an ideal dinner for those following AIP, offering deep flavors and a satisfying meal.

Ingredients:

- 4 salmon fillets
- 2 tbsp olive oil
- 1 tsp lemon juice
- 1 tsp garlic powder
- 1 tsp fresh thyme
- 2 carrots, peeled and sliced
- 1 sweet potato, peeled and diced
- 1 small parsnip, peeled and sliced
- Salt and pepper to taste

Instructions:

1. Preheat your oven to 400°F (200°C).
2. In a bowl, toss the sliced carrots, sweet potato, and parsnip with olive oil, salt, and pepper. Arrange them on a baking sheet in a single layer.
3. Roast vegetables for 25-30 minutes, stirring halfway through, until tender and lightly browned.
4. While the vegetables are roasting, prepare the salmon. Drizzle the salmon fillets with olive oil, lemon juice, and sprinkle with garlic powder and thyme.

5. Place the salmon fillets on a separate baking sheet and bake for 12–15 minutes or until cooked through.
6. Serve the roasted root vegetables with the baked salmon and enjoy a nutrient-packed, delicious meal.

These meal options and recipes are just a few of the many ways you can incorporate the Autoimmune Protocol into your daily life. With a focus on whole, anti-inflammatory foods, these meals will nourish your body while helping to manage and heal autoimmune conditions.

Snacks and Beverages

Snacks and beverages are essential for staying energized and satisfied between meals, especially when following the Autoimmune Protocol (AIP). However, many conventional snacks and drinks contain inflammatory ingredients that can hinder the healing process. To make your AIP journey easier and more enjoyable, the following snack and beverage ideas are both delicious and nourishing, designed to fuel your body while supporting your autoimmune health.

1. AIP Veggie Chips

These homemade vegetable chips are a crunchy, satisfying snack that can be easily customized based on your preferences. Rich in fiber, antioxidants, and healthy fats, they're perfect for when you're craving something salty and crispy.

Ingredients:

- 2 sweet potatoes, thinly sliced
- 1 zucchini, thinly sliced
- 1 tbsp olive oil

- 1 tsp sea salt
- 1 tsp garlic powder
- 1 tsp rosemary (optional)

Instructions:

1. Preheat your oven to 375°F (190°C).
2. Place the sliced vegetables on a baking sheet and drizzle with olive oil. Toss to coat.
3. Sprinkle with sea salt, garlic powder, and rosemary (if using).
4. Bake for 20-25 minutes, flipping halfway through, until the chips are crispy and golden.
5. Allow them to cool slightly before serving.

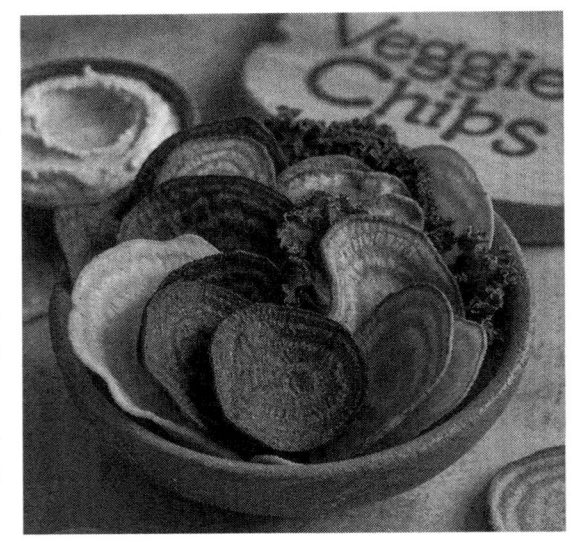

2. AIP Guacamole with Carrot and Cucumber Sticks

Guacamole is a flavorful, nutrient-dense snack that's rich in healthy fats, making it a perfect choice for the AIP. Pair it with fresh vegetable sticks for a satisfying and crunchy snack.

Ingredients:

- 2 ripe avocados, mashed
- 1 tbsp fresh lime juice
- 1 tbsp fresh cilantro, chopped
- 1 small cucumber, sliced into sticks

- 2 carrots, peeled and cut into sticks
- A pinch of salt

Instructions:

1. In a bowl, mash the avocados and mix with lime juice and cilantro.
2. Season with a pinch of salt.
3. Serve the guacamole with the cucumber and carrot sticks for dipping.

3. AIP Energy Bites

These no-bake energy bites are a fantastic source of healthy fats, protein, and fiber. They're perfect for an afternoon snack or when you need a quick pick-me-up.

Ingredients:

- 1 cup unsweetened shredded coconut
- 2 tbsp coconut oil
- 2 tbsp sunflower seeds (or pumpkin seeds)
- 1 tbsp raw honey (optional)
- 1 tsp vanilla extract
- Pinch of sea salt

Instructions:

1. In a food processor, pulse together the shredded coconut, sunflower seeds, and sea salt until finely ground.
2. Add coconut oil, honey (optional), and vanilla extract. Process until the mixture sticks together.
3. Roll the mixture into small bite-sized balls.
4. Refrigerate for at least an hour to firm up before serving.

4. AIP Apple Cinnamon Muffins

These light and fluffy muffins make a perfect snack, providing natural sweetness from apples while still being completely compliant with the AIP.

Ingredients:

- 2 apples, peeled, cored, and grated
- 2 cups coconut flour
- 1 tbsp ground cinnamon
- 2 eggs
- 1/4 cup coconut oil, melted
- 1 tbsp maple syrup (optional)
- 1 tsp baking soda
- 1/4 cup water

Instructions:

1. Preheat your oven to 350°F (175°C) and line a muffin tin with paper liners.
2. In a large bowl, combine coconut flour, cinnamon, and baking soda.
3. In another bowl, whisk together eggs, melted coconut oil, maple syrup, and water.
4. Add the grated apples and wet ingredients to the dry ingredients. Stir to combine.
5. Pour the batter into the muffin tin and bake for 20-25 minutes or until a toothpick comes out clean.

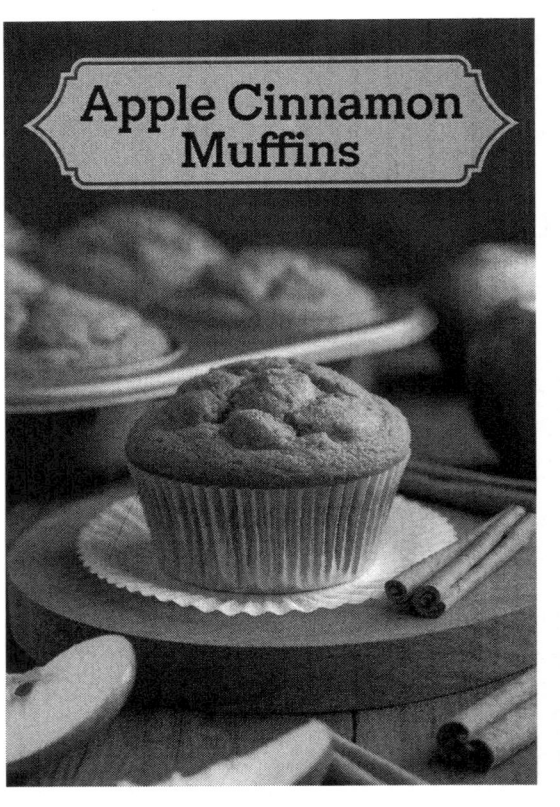

5. AIP Bone Broth

Bone broth is a nourishing beverage that is rich in collagen, gelatin, and essential amino acids, making it a healing drink for the gut and joints. It's a comforting drink that can be enjoyed throughout the day.

Ingredients:

- 2 lbs of grass-fed beef or chicken bones (or a mix)
- 1 onion, quartered
- 3 garlic cloves, smashed
- 2 carrots, chopped
- 2 celery stalks, chopped
- 1 tbsp apple cider vinegar
- 1 tsp sea salt
- Water to cover

Instructions:

1. Place the bones, vegetables, apple cider vinegar, and sea salt in a large pot or slow cooker.
2. Cover with water and bring to a boil.
3. Reduce the heat to low and let the broth simmer for at least 12 hours (24 hours for richer flavor).
4. Once done, strain the broth and store it in jars or containers.
5. Sip the warm broth as a soothing, nutrient-packed beverage.

Desserts and Treats

Satisfying your sweet tooth while following the Autoimmune Protocol can be challenging, but it's entirely possible to enjoy healthy, AIP-friendly desserts. These treats are made with natural, whole ingredients that nourish the body and keep inflammation at bay. Whether you're in the mood for something fruity, creamy, or chocolatey, these desserts offer a delicious way to indulge without compromising your health.

1. AIP Chocolate Avocado Pudding

This creamy, rich chocolate pudding is made with ripe avocados for a velvety texture, combined with AIP-compliant ingredients to provide a naturally sweet, indulgent dessert without refined sugar or dairy.

Ingredients:

- 2 ripe avocados, peeled and pitted
- 1/4 cup raw cacao powder
- 2 tbsp maple syrup (optional)
- 1 tsp vanilla extract
- 1/4 cup coconut milk
- Pinch of sea salt

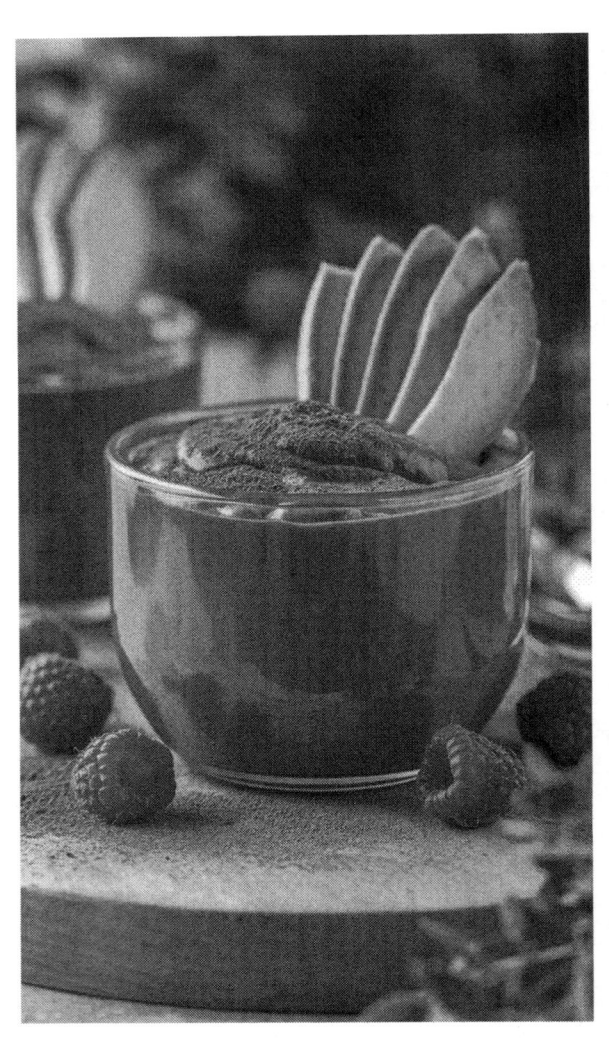

Instructions:

1. Place all ingredients in a blender or food processor.

2. Blend until smooth and creamy, scraping down the sides as needed.
3. Taste and adjust sweetness by adding more maple syrup if desired.
4. Chill the pudding for at least 30 minutes before serving.
5. Garnish with fresh berries or a sprinkle of coconut flakes for extra flavor.

2. AIP Coconut Mango Sorbet

This tropical sorbet is refreshing, fruity, and incredibly easy to make. Made with coconut milk and mango, it's a guilt-free treat that's perfect for warm weather.

Ingredients:

- 2 ripe mangoes, peeled and chopped
- 1 cup coconut milk (full-fat, unsweetened)
- 1 tbsp fresh lime juice
- 1 tbsp raw honey (optional)

Instructions:

1. In a blender, combine mango, coconut milk, lime juice, and honey (optional).
2. Blend until smooth.
3. Pour the mixture into a shallow container and freeze for at least 4 hours, or until solid.
4. Before serving, let the sorbet sit at room temperature for a few minutes to soften slightly.
5. Scoop into bowls and enjoy!

3. AIP Apple Cinnamon Crisps

These baked apple chips are a naturally sweet and crunchy dessert. With a touch of cinnamon, they offer a warm, comforting flavor that satisfies your dessert cravings.

Ingredients:

- 2 large apples, thinly sliced
- 1 tsp cinnamon
- 1 tsp vanilla extract (optional)

Instructions:

1. Preheat your oven to 250°F (120°C) and line a baking sheet with parchment paper.
2. Arrange the apple slices in a single layer on the baking sheet.
3. Sprinkle with cinnamon and drizzle with vanilla extract, if using.
4. Bake for 1.5–2 hours, flipping halfway through, until the apples are crispy and golden.
5. Allow the chips to cool before serving.

4. AIP Chocolate Dipped Strawberries

These chocolate-dipped strawberries are a simple yet elegant dessert that provides a dose of antioxidants and healthy fats, making them a great choice for a sweet treat.

Ingredients:

- 10 strawberries, washed and dried
- 1/4 cup coconut oil

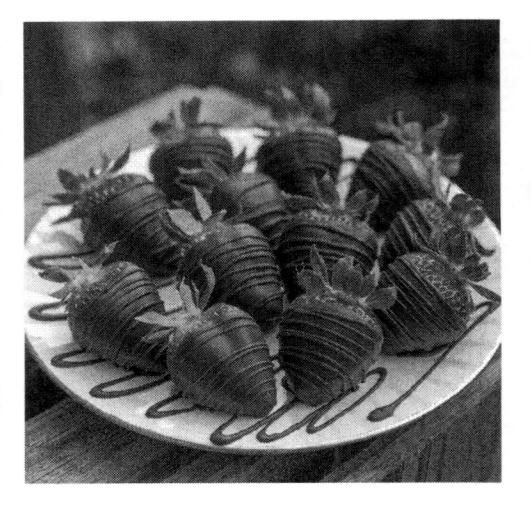

- 2 tbsp raw cacao powder
- 1 tbsp maple syrup (optional)

Instructions:

1. Melt the coconut oil in a small saucepan over low heat.
2. Stir in raw cacao powder and maple syrup (optional). Mix until smooth.
3. Dip each strawberry into the chocolate mixture and place it on a parchment-lined tray.
4. Refrigerate for 30 minutes to allow the chocolate to harden.
5. Serve and enjoy!

Weekly Meal Plans and Shopping Lists

Creating a weekly meal plan that adheres to the Autoimmune Protocol (AIP) can feel daunting at first, but with a little organization and preparation, it can become second nature. By following a structured meal plan, you ensure that you're consistently eating foods that support healing, while avoiding potential triggers that may exacerbate autoimmune conditions. The following weekly meal plan provides a variety of nutrient-dense meals that cater to the AIP, along with a comprehensive shopping list to help streamline your grocery store trips.

Week 1 Meal Plan

Day 1

Breakfast: AIP Scrambled Eggs with Avocado and Sautéed Spinach
Lunch: Grilled Chicken Salad with Mixed Greens, Carrots, and Olive Oil Vinaigrette
Dinner: Baked Salmon with Roasted Sweet Potatoes and Steamed Broccoli
Snack: AIP Coconut Mango Sorbet

Day 2

Breakfast: AIP Banana Pancakes with Coconut Whipped Cream
Lunch: Turkey Lettuce Wraps with Cucumber, Avocado, and AIP Mayo
Dinner: Zucchini Noodles with AIP Meatballs and Tomato-Free Marinara
Snack: Sliced Apple with AIP Pumpkin Seed Butter

Day 3

Breakfast: AIP Smoothie (Coconut Milk, Blueberries, Spinach, and Collagen Protein)
Lunch: Sweet Potato and Kale Soup with Grass-Fed Beef
Dinner: Herb-Roasted Chicken with Carrot Fries and Garlic-Infused Olive Oil
Snack: AIP Energy Bites

Day 4

Breakfast: AIP Pumpkin Muffins with Chia Seeds
Lunch: Grilled Shrimp Salad with Mixed Greens and Lemon Dressing
Dinner: Slow Cooker Beef Stew with Root Vegetables
Snack: AIP Veggie Chips with Guacamole

Day 5

Breakfast: AIP Egg-Free Apple Cinnamon Pancakes
Lunch: Roasted Chicken with Cabbage Slaw and Olive Oil
Dinner: Baked Cod with Roasted Brussels Sprouts and Sweet Potato Mash
Snack: Fresh Berries with AIP Coconut Yogurt

Day 6

Breakfast: AIP Porridge (Made with Coconut Flour, Chia Seeds, and Cinnamon)
Lunch: AIP Turkey Meatballs with Cauliflower Rice
Dinner: Grilled Steak with Steamed Asparagus and Zucchini
Snack: Carrot and Celery Sticks with AIP-friendly Sunflower Seed Butter

Day 7

Breakfast: AIP Breakfast Sausages with Roasted Sweet Potatoes and Avocado
Lunch: AIP Tuna Salad Lettuce Wraps with Sliced Cucumbers
Dinner: Grilled Lamb Chops with Garlic Mashed Cauliflower and Steamed Kale
Snack: AIP Chocolate-Dipped Strawberries

Weekly Shopping List

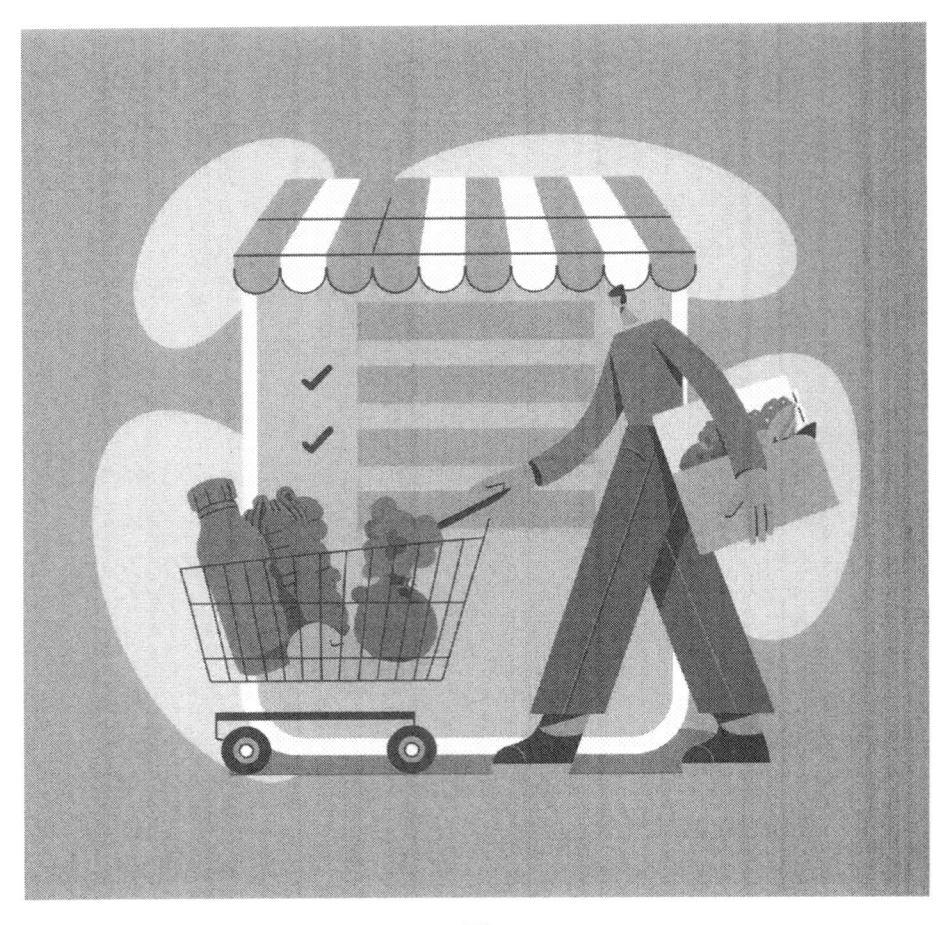

This shopping list contains the core ingredients you'll need for the week's meals. Always try to purchase organic, grass-fed, and pasture-raised options when possible to ensure maximum nutrition and quality.

Proteins

- Grass-fed beef (ground, stew meat, steaks)
- Skinless chicken breasts and thighs
- Salmon fillets
- Shrimp
- Grass-fed lamb chops
- Eggs (pasture-raised)
- Tuna (canned in water, no additives)
- Collagen protein powder (AIP-friendly)

Vegetables

- Sweet potatoes
- Carrots
- Zucchini
- Kale
- Broccoli
- Brussels sprouts
- Asparagus
- Spinach
- Mixed greens (such as arugula, kale, and spinach)
- Cabbage
- Cauliflower (for mash and rice)
- Cucumbers
- Garlic
- Onion
- Fresh herbs (parsley, cilantro, rosemary, thyme)

Fruits

- Avocados
- Apples
- Bananas
- Blueberries (fresh or frozen)
- Mangoes (fresh or frozen)
- Strawberries (fresh or frozen)
- Lemons
- Limes

Healthy Fats

- Olive oil (extra virgin)
- Coconut oil
- Coconut milk (full-fat, unsweetened)
- Sunflower seed butter
- Pumpkin seed butter
- Chia seeds
- Raw coconut flakes
- Cacao butter (optional for desserts)

Dairy Alternatives

- AIP coconut yogurt (unsweetened)
- Coconut milk (for smoothies, soups, and curries)

Pantry Staples

- Coconut flour
- Almond flour (AIP-friendly)
- Apple cider vinegar
- Raw honey (for sweetening, optional)
- Maple syrup (for sweetening, optional)
- Sea salt
- Ground cinnamon
- Ground ginger
- Raw cacao powder (for desserts and smoothies)
- Collagen powder
- Gelatin (for AIP jellies or gummies)

AIP Condiments and Spices

- AIP mayonnaise
- AIP-approved mustard
- AIP-friendly spice blends (without nightshades)
- Rosemary
- Basil
- Thyme
- Oregano
- Garlic powder (nightshade-free)
- Onion powder
- Turmeric

Tips for Meal Prep and Shopping

1. **Batch Cooking**: Prepare larger portions of soups, stews, or meats and freeze them in individual servings to reduce the amount of cooking during the week.
2. **Pre-cut Vegetables**: Wash, peel, and chop your vegetables at the start of the week to make meal prep quicker and easier.
3. **Use Leftovers**: Leftover meat or vegetables from one meal can easily be repurposed into salads or soups for the next day's meals.
4. **Snack Prep**: Pre-portion AIP-friendly snacks such as veggie chips, energy bites, and fruits to have easy grab-and-go options throughout the week.
5. **Shopping Strategy**: Stick to the perimeter of the grocery store where the fresh produce, meat, and dairy alternatives are located. Avoid processed foods typically found in the center aisles.

By following this weekly meal plan and shopping list, you'll have all the ingredients you need to maintain a nutrient-rich, AIP-compliant diet that supports your autoimmune healing journey. Planning ahead helps reduce stress and makes it easier to stay consistent with your health goals.

Conclusion

A New Path to Healing and Wellness

As you reach the end of *The Autoimmune Protocol*, it's important to reflect on the transformative journey you are about to embark on. Whether you're struggling with an autoimmune disease or simply seeking better overall health, the power to heal lies within your grasp. The protocols and strategies outlined in this book are not just a diet—they are a path to a new way of living, one that is grounded in nourishing your body, healing your gut, and addressing the root causes of inflammation that fuel autoimmune conditions.

This book has shared with you the scientific foundations of autoimmune diseases, the science behind the Autoimmune Protocol (AIP), and the real-world applications of the elimination and reintroduction phases. You've learned about the foods to embrace, those to avoid, and how each phase works to restore balance in the body. By now, you also understand the critical importance of lifestyle factors—such as stress management, sleep, exercise, and community support—that enhance the effectiveness of AIP and help you maintain long-term success.

Adopting the Autoimmune Protocol is not a quick fix; it's a commitment to restoring your health for the long term. It's a powerful tool for addressing the underlying causes of autoimmune diseases, helping you regain control of your life. As you follow the steps laid out in this book, remember that healing is a process. Some days may be challenging, but each step you take brings you closer to the vibrant, healthy life you deserve.

Key Takeaways from the Book:

- **Personalized Healing:** The Autoimmune Protocol offers a unique, tailored approach to healing that focuses on addressing the root causes of autoimmune conditions through diet and lifestyle changes.
- **Patience and Persistence:** Healing takes time. The AIP process may be demanding, but the results speak for themselves—improved symptoms, restored energy, and a renewed sense of vitality.
- **Community and Support:** Surround yourself with a community of like-minded individuals, whether online or in person, who are on a similar healing journey. The power of shared experiences and support cannot be overstated.
- **Self-Awareness and Adaptability:** Listen to your body, adjust your protocol as needed, and be flexible. Each person's healing journey is unique, and there's no "one-size-fits-all" approach.

If you've made it this far, you've already taken the most important step—committing to a healthier, more empowered version of yourself. Continue to explore, experiment, and adapt as you fine-tune your path to healing. Remember that your journey is just beginning, and with the knowledge, tools, and mindset shared in this book, you have everything you need to thrive.

Finally, know that healing is not just about the absence of disease. It's about reclaiming your life, your vitality, and your health—something that the Autoimmune Protocol offers in abundance. As you move forward, take pride in the progress you've made, knowing that you are on the path to lasting wellness. Your body has an incredible ability to heal. Let the Autoimmune Protocol guide you to a future free from the limitations of autoimmune disease, and embrace the vibrant life that awaits you.

Wishing you health, vitality, and joy on your healing journey.

Printed in Great Britain
by Amazon